How to Successfully Become a Vegetarian

How to Successfully Become a Vegetarian

Rudy Hadisentosa

Copyright 2009

Rudy hadisentosa

ISBN: 978-0-557-08768-6

Introduction

If you don't have the time to read the whole book but are interested in becoming a vegetarian, here's what this book does:

It gives you strong enough reason to actually become a vegetarian, without complaining and without ever looking back at your previous lifestyle. You will know in your heart that every time you see meat, you will just not want it anymore. Even when friends try to tempt you, you will not be interested. You will have no more cravings. Instead, you will be far happier with your vegetarian diet. You will become a life-long vegetarian.

This book was written in a way that connects with your heart; it explains all the reasons why you should go vegetarian. You will be able to conquer every hurdle that you encounter in your transition process. You will also know for certain why you want to change your lifestyle. And this is crucial because *if you don't know why you want to become a vegetarian, you will fail. That's for sure*. Actually, that's the biggest reason why so many people go back to their previous lifestyle. They try being vegetarian, meet little challenges, can't handle them, and then decide to quit. They say to themselves, "Okay, why am I doing this? Let's call it a day." Actually, these people don't have their *own reasoning* to go vegetarian.

And this is where this book plays its part: to help you find your *own reasoning* to go vegetarian in a way that you would not trade your new lifestyle for anything.

Your must find your own reasoning in your heart or else you will fail. So let's find it together.

Table of Contents

CHAPTER 1:	Pesco, Ovo-Lacto, Vegan—Defining the Types of Vegetarians	1
CHAPTER 2:	A Brief History of Vegetarianism—How It Started and What It All Means	7
CHAPTER 3:	Ethical Eating—Why Becoming a Vegetarian Is Good for You and for the Earth	19
CHAPTER 4:	Where Do I Begin? Getting Started on Your Meatless Journey	33
CHAPTER 5:	Vegetarian Nutrition—Getting Everything Your Body Needs	49
CHAPTER 6:	Parasites—The Guests Who Came to Dinner	65
CHAPTER 7:	The Happy Vegetarian—How a Meatless Diet Will Improve Your Health and Well-Being	73
CHAPTER 8:	"But I'm Not a Freak!" or, "How Do I Cope in a Carnivorous World?"	83
CHAPTER 9:	The Vegetarian Eats Out—Meals You Can Enjoy, from Fast Food to Fine Dining	99
CHAPTER 10:	Balancing the Scales—Losing Weight while on a Vegetarian Diet	111
CHAPTER 11:	Exercising the Mind, Body, and Spirit—Vegetarian Style	123
CHAPTER 12:	The Meatless Kitchen—Buying Food and Planning Menus	129

Chapter 13:	Delicious Vegetarian Recipes that Everyone Can Enjoy	143
Chapter 14:	Shopping in the Health Food Aisle—Solving the Mysteries of Seeds, Soy, and Stevia	153
Chapter 15:	The Pros and Cons of Milk, Cheese, Yogurt, and Other Dairy Products	169
Chapter 16:	Special Needs—How to Live a Meatless Life and Still Make Your Doctor (or Coach) Happy	179
Chapter 17:	Veggies for Kids—How to Raise a Happy, Healthy Vegetarian Child	191
Chapter 18:	The Social Vegetarian—Connecting with Meat Eaters and Others at Work and at Play	199
Chapter 19:	How to Create a Vegetarian—Supportive Environment in Your Home and Office	207
Chapter 20:	Ethics, Beauty, and Health—Saving the Earth, One Veggie Burger at a Time	215
Chapter 21:	The Path Ahead—Enjoying Your Vegetarian Lifestyle for the Rest of Your Life	225
Chapter 22:	FAQ—Finding the Answers to the Most Commonly Asked Questions about Vegetarianism	233

CHAPTER 1
Pesco, Ovo-Lacto, Vegan
Defining the Types of Vegetarians

To most nonvegetarians, the vegetarian lifestyle is mysterious and confusing. They have a hard time visualizing what a vegetarian's plate of food might look like. To nonvegetarians, the plate looks empty and unappetizing as they imagine it filled with leaves of lettuce and radishes. Of course, vegetarians eat a variety of plant-based foods besides lettuce and radishes. Still, the meat eater remains puzzled, and numerous questions often arise in his mind. Do vegetarians totally shun animal protein? Does that include eggs and milk? Is it something they do for health reasons or because they love animals? And how do they get enough protein in their diets if they don't eat meat? Relax. Take a deep breath. The answers to these burning questions (and many others) will most likely be answered in this book. We just need to take it one step at a time, starting with the definition of a vegetarian.

According to the dictionary, a vegetarian is defined as "a person who does not eat meat, and sometimes other animal products, especially for moral, religious, or health reasons." However, if you take a poll of vegetarians, you'd quickly discover that there are almost as many ways to be a vegetarian as there are, well, vegetarians. Some people claim to be vegetarians when really they've just cut back on the amount of animal products they consume. On the other end of the scale, there are vegetarians who eat no animal protein at all, or anything produced by animals—such as milk, eggs, and honey. So the first thing to consider when approaching the vegetarian lifestyle is exactly what kind of vegetarian you plan to be.

Vegetarian Diets—the Big Three

There are three main vegetarian diets, although variations abound in each category: ovo-lacto-vegetarian, lacto-vegetarian, and vegan. Let's take them one at a time and look at the differences:

An ovo-lacto-vegetarian diet means eating mostly plant foods, but also having eggs and dairy products including yogurt, milk, cheese, and ice cream. This is the first step most people take when they switch to a vegetarian diet, because it's easy to fulfill all your nutritional requirements and, well, everything tastes good when you cover it with cheese! It's also an easy diet to maintain in the real world, as there are always restaurant choices—including fast-food options—so no matter where you are or who you're with, you can always find something to eat.

Lacto-vegetarians eat no animal protein or eggs; instead they consume dairy products. While acceptable dairy substitutes have become much more palatable in recent years, it can still be difficult to avoid dairy entirely; this makes cooking much more challenging. Many lacto-vegetarians don't eat eggs because, as a growing ovum, they're potentially animals. Or they choose not to eat eggs because they're uncomfortable with egg-farming practices. Conversely, there are ovo-vegetarians, who eat eggs but don't consume dairy products.

Vegans eschew all animal proteins and animal by-products. This is the most extreme form of vegetarian diet, as vegans get all of their nutrition from grains, vegetables, fruits, legumes, nuts, and seeds. And vegans must avoid a large number of commercially produced foods that contain animal proteins; most breads are made with eggs, for example, and many nondairy products are thickened with casein, a protein extracted from milk. Even vegetarian burgers often contain eggs! It can be difficult in today's society to maintain a vegan lifestyle. But simply educating yourself on where, when, and what animal products are being used can make all the difference. Learning about alternatives to animal products is especially useful. Most animal rights groups will have information available for you to use. Despite the challenges, the vegan diet has steadily grown in popularity in recent years as more and more vegetarians have become savvy label readers and vegan-friendly food companies have created more products for them to enjoy.

In addition to the three basic vegetarian diets, there's also macrobiotics, a diet inspired by the ancient Chinese principle of yin and yang, which relies primarily on locally produced, seasonal foods. The basic macrobiotic diet includes fish. Remove the fish and the diet is vegan, with most macrobiotic cookbooks heavily favoring Asian-influenced cuisine and the use of ingredients like pickled vegetables, daikon radishes, and sea vegetables like kelp and nori.

This isn't to say that you're required to sign up for any one style of vegetarian diet and follow it to the letter. Pesco vegetarians, for example, don't eat poultry, beef, or pork, but they do eat fish. (Fish offer many nutrients, including omega-3.) The so-called semivegetarians have cut back on their intake of meat overall, but they still eat it occasionally—if you're reading this, that's probably where you are already! Pollo vegetarians avoid red meat and fish but eat chicken, while the pesco-pollo vegetarians avoid red meat but consume both chicken and fish. There are even fruitarians, who only eat seeds, nuts, and fruit, plus vegetables that are botanically classified as fruit like zucchini, eggplant, squash, and avocados. And there are other diets that, while vegetarian in nature, further restrict consumption of certain foods depending on the diet's purpose—the raw food diet requires that you only eat uncooked foods, and the natural-hygiene diet, while making limited use of animal products, is designed to cleanse the body of toxins and chooses the allowed foods accordingly.

But don't let all of that confuse you. As a newcomer to vegetarianism, you should first set your sights on the three primary types of the vegetarian diet: ovo-lacto, lacto, and vegan. Once you've discovered which of these best meets your needs, you can decide if you want to adapt them even further, adding or subtracting as you see fit. For the most part, labeling your diet is less important than figuring out how to transition from a nonvegetarian diet to a vegetarian one. Remember, becoming a vegetarian is an evolutionary process. It doesn't happen overnight. Adopting a new mind-set when it comes to food and how you eat it takes time. Be patient and enjoy the journey.

Which Comes First, the Dairy Product or the Egg?

Giving up meat but holding onto eggs and dairy products in your diet is a good way to start your vegetarian experience. Your menu options are far greater, and it's easier to work enough protein into your diet than jumping straight to a macrobiotic or vegan lifestyle. Yes, there are good reasons to avoid eggs and dairy, and we'll discuss that as we go along. But ovo-lacto-vegetarianism is perhaps the most popular, simple, and straightforward approach to vegetarianism.

Besides being a great protein source, eggs also provide your body with lecithin, a substance that emulsifies dietary fat and is needed to build cell walls. In fact, lecithin is very important in protecting your cells from oxidation and is vital in building the protective tissues that surround the brain. (Should you choose not to eat eggs, lecithin is still important; but there are now lecithin supplements that have been shown to improve blood cholesterol levels.)

Eggs are an easy meal and, for many vegetarians, the veggie omelet is a great fallback meal that's available at virtually every coffee shop. You should limit the amount of yolks you eat, though, as they're high in fat and cholesterol; egg whites, on the other hand, are almost pure protein.

As for dairy products, you may find yourself going overboard when you first start your vegetarian diet, making up for the loss of meat by eating more cheese and drinking more milk. Keep an eye on the amount of fat you're eating; changing your diet isn't going to make you feel better if you start loading up on extra fat and cholesterol!

So … What Can I Have for Lunch?

If your first thought is that you're about to embark on a way of eating that's going to be boring, repetitive, and limiting, then you have a surprise in store. Vegetarians—vegans included—enjoy a widely varied diet made up of tasty and nutritious foods, most of which you already eat on a regular basis.

All of the same things that you eat today—burritos, burgers, casseroles, soups, lasagna, sandwiches—can be enjoyed as part of a vegetarian diet. All you need to do is remove or replace the meat. The key is to make sure you get enough protein from combining grains and legumes (which we'll discuss in detail in chapter 5) and choose your meals wisely.

Take that burrito, for example. Skip the nonvegetarian style, and go for one that's packed with beans, rice, tomatoes, onions, bell peppers, and sour cream. It's chock-full of protein and other vital nutrients and is absolutely delicious. Even something as decadent as Stroganoff can be adapted to a meat-free diet—cubes of Portobello mushrooms, marinated in soy sauce, make for a fine meat substitute when tossed with noodles, spices, and cream.

And don't overlook the cuisine of cultures that have long celebrated vegetarian cooking. Miso soup, Spanikopita, hummus, vegetable curries, tabbouleh salad, samosas, and veggie stir-fry dishes are all on your menu—so enjoy!

Once you become accustomed to eating vegetarian meals, you'll find that it's much easier than you think. With a little creativity, you can even plan entire meatless dinner parties around foods so delicious that your most carnivorous guests won't even notice that meat is missing from the menu—a dinner of hearty vegetable chili topped with shredded cheese and a spring salad of field greens, toasted walnuts, and crumbled bleu cheese in a balsamic vinaigrette, followed by key lime pie for dessert ... well, who wouldn't love that?

By choosing to adopt the vegetarian lifestyle, you're going to improve your health, help conserve the earth's natural resources, eat more ethically and responsibly, and lower your risk of contracting meat-borne illnesses from E. coli contamination and additives like hormones, chemicals, and antibiotics. But that doesn't mean your diet has to be boring; there's a whole world of foods out there that you can enjoy!

Whatever the reason you've decided to remove meat from your diet, you'll find that it's the best nutritional decision that you've ever made. In the course of this book, you'll learn about the fascinating history of vegetarianism, how you can transition from a nonvegetarian diet to a vegetarian one, the ways in which you can ensure that you're getting proper nutrition, how to buy food and cook for your family, and how to stick with your diet in a world full of carnivores.

You're about to embark on a journey that will make you healthier and happier. Congratulations on choosing to live as a thoughtful, caring eater; your body (and the earth) will thank you!

CHAPTER 2

A Brief History of Vegetarianism
How It Started and What It All Means

When you think of early man, odds are that the first image that pops into your mind is that of a spear-carrying Neanderthal dragging a large, dead animal home to his cave for dinner. We've long held onto the erroneous notion that our ancestors were mighty warriors who took down gigantic beasts with their bows, arrows, and flint knives, and tore into meat as their primary source of nourishment.

But the truth is more complicated than that. Certainly there were eras in human history when meat was a staple; during the Ice Age, for example, the ground was so cold and hard that there was hardly any vegetation, so the Neanderthal was forced to hunt down animals to fill his grumbling tummy. But the very earliest humans were more gatherers than hunters and actually scavenged the remains of animals that were killed by other predators. Studies by anthropologists indicate that early man was far more interested in feasting on the nutrient-rich bone marrow of animals rather than on their flesh and that he used tools to cut away the meat, not to eat it, but to remove it from the desired bones.

Early man's diet consisted of what he could find growing where he lived— vegetables, fruits, nuts, and seeds. By combining those, and relying primarily on a diet of calcium-rich wild greens, he was able to get all of the vitamins, iron, protein, fats, and carbohydrates that he needed. Animals were yet to be domesticated, so the only meat our ancestors had to eat was either what they chased down or found lying about—gathering nuts and seeds was simply more productive than counting on being able to catch and cook an animal by supper time. Eventually, man developed agriculture, raising vegetables and grains and domesticating animals for meat and dairy. But, before that time, some ten thousand years ago, man relied heavily on that which he could pluck from trees, bushes, and the ground, and 90 percent of his diet was made up of plant food. So toss out the idea that man is at heart a carnivore; we are, in fact, omnivores, able to eat meat but certainly not required to by our biology or our history.

The Pythagorean Credo

By the time man's adventures were being jotted down in scriptures and testaments, nonvegetarians had become commonplace, but there were still those who advised against the practice. In the Old Testament's Book of Daniel, it is said that Daniel refused the wealthy king Nebuchadnezzar's feast of rich foods, meat, and wine and asked for only vegetables and water for ten days. At the end of that period, Daniel asked that his health and that of his companions be compared to those who indulged in the fare of the king's table, and Daniel's group was deemed "better in appearance and fatter in flesh" than those who ate the king's diet. The parable was intended to show that Daniel was a smart, strong iconoclast, able to assert himself in the presence of a king, but it also serves as one of the earliest records of the superiority of a vegetarian lifestyle—and how going against the nonvegetarian norm was, even then, considered an act of rebellion!

But the earliest vegetarian diet, way back in the sixth century BC and long before the term "vegetarian" was coined, was the Pythagorean Diet. The Greek philosopher Pythagoras, famous for his contributions to geometry and mathematics, strongly believed in the reincarnation of the soul; he preached an ethical lifestyle that included injunctions against killing living creatures, whether for purpose of sacrifice or for eating of meat. His prescribed diet was very close to today's vegan diet and attracted two different classes of adherents. One elite group, who studied directly under Pythagoras and was called the *mathematikoi* ("mathematicians"), followed an extremely restricted regimen, eating only cereals, bread, honey, fruits, and some vegetables. A larger group of followers, who attended lectures by the philosopher and was called the *akousmatikoi* ("listeners"), were allowed to eat meat and drink wine but were required to abstain on certain days.

According to historical documents, Pythagoras told his followers, "Oh, my fellow men! Do not defile your bodies with sinful foods. We have corn, we have apples bending down the branches with their weight, and we have grapes swelling on the vines. There are sweet herbs, and vegetables, which can be cooked and softened over the fire, nor are you denied milk or thyme-scented honey. The earth affords a lavish supply of riches, of innocent foods, and offers you banquets that involve no bloodshed or slaughter: only beasts satisfy their hunger with flesh, and not even all of those, because horses, cattle, and sheep live on grass." His biographer, Diogenes, wrote that Pythagoras ate millet or barley bread and honeycomb in the morning and raw vegetables at night and that he paid fishermen to throw their catches back into the ocean.

The Pythagorean diet—which the philosopher claimed the goddess Demeter had taught to Heracles who in turn had taught the same to him—became known as the choice of intellectuals and rebels and was banned by the Roman government. But in the smaller, outlying Greek states, the Pythagorean diet was more acceptable and found a wide share of adherents. Pythagoras wasn't the only philosopher to advise that a vegetarian diet was healthier and more ethical than a meat-eating one. Hippocrates, Socrates, Plato, Seneca, Ovid, and Virgil, all advocated vegetarian diets. Throughout the times that followed, Pythagoras' teachings, including his diet, retained its advocates, even seeing a resurgence of popularity in Europe during the seventeenth century when a devout Christian named Thomas Tryon read the works of the German mystic Jacob Böhme and started a Hindu vegetarian society in London.

Toward an Enlightened Way of Eating

The Age of Enlightenment during Europe's eighteenth century saw an upsurge in interest in vegetarianism following hundreds of years in which diet was dictated by need; after all, during periods of famine and disease, one eats whatever one can get. But by the eighteenth century, medicine had curtailed many of the more widespread diseases, and Europeans had discovered a number of delicious New World vegetables like potatoes, cauliflower, and corn. The intellectuals of the time—including the philosopher Arthur Schopenhauer who started thinking about loftier issues than mere survival—began to reappraise man's place in the order of things. For the first time, arguments were put forth that animals were intelligent, feeling creatures and that it was immoral to kill or mistreat them.

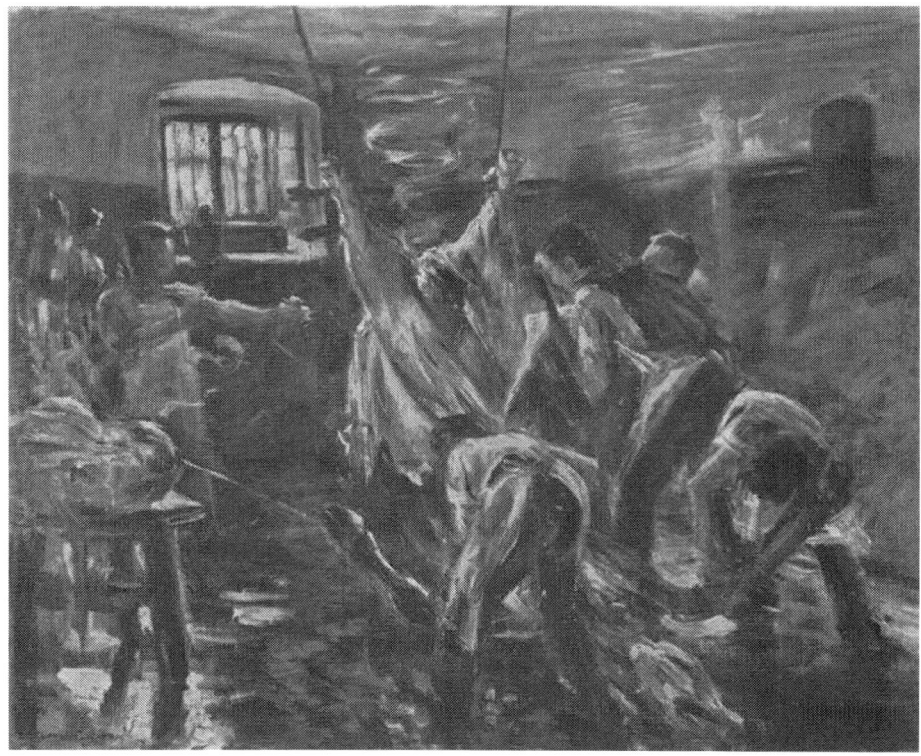

During the eighteenth century, painters like Oudry and Delacroix made artworks that showed animals as individuals with personalities rather than just beasts to be used and slaughtered for human convenience. During this time, the treatment of animals was often horrific; beating one's horse wasn't considered reprehensible, neither were cockfights, bear baiting, or the setting of bulldogs against bears for sport. Pigs were beaten to death with knotted ropes in the belief that it would make for more tender meat; in Paris, the slaughter of animals was done in the alleys next to the city's butcher shops, and this led to public outcry against the horrible sounds of slaughter, the blood in the streets, and the stench of rotting flesh. When Napoleon took control of Paris in 1799, he began a program of extensive city works that included construction of sewers and slaughterhouses on the outskirts of the city. The methods used to butcher animals remained the same, but at least people no longer had to witness the slaughter as they walked down the city streets; thus began the tradition of mass killing of animals for meat behind closed doors that continues to this day.

The 1800s saw the emergence of a number of religious and educational communities which advocated vegetarian diets. In 1807, Reverend William Cowherd broke with the Church of England and established the Bible Christian Church; it was founded on a literal interpretation of the scriptures. Cowherd believed that the Bible prohibited the eating of meat—a view that was not shared by leaders of the Church of England—and he quickly developed a large congregation. His timing was perfect; he capitalized on a widespread backlash to the industrial revolution that inspired a more romanticized view of nature and animals. Cowherd's flock abstained from consuming meat, coffee, tea, tobacco, and alcohol, and many also eschewed dairy products and eggs. The Bible Christian Church handed out free bowls of vegetable soup to the poor, and it is often credited with coining the term "vegetarian."

In 1817, a disciple of Cowherd's named William Metcalfe sailed for America with forty-one church members and formed a small but influential Philadelphia congregation. Among Metcalfe's followers was a Presbyterian minister named Sylvester Graham, a raw foods enthusiast and inventor of the graham cracker. Graham toured the United States, giving lectures on temperance (abstinence from alcohol) and the importance of proper diet to sustain good health. Through his lectures and his writings in the *Graham Journal of Health and Longevity,* he counseled that certain foods, such as white bread and alcohol, and activities, such as the wearing of tight pants, were unhealthy because of their "stimulating" qualities. He was a tireless advocate of the vegetarian diet and founded the American Vegetarian Society in 1850; he compared human physiology to that of orangutans, concluding that vegetarian food was optimal for all primates. He lectured extensively on the connection between diet and disease, stating that New York residents had weakened their resistance to epidemics through their unhealthy eating habits. He promoted the use of whole grains, denouncing the increasingly popular use of refined flour in baked foods and pointing out that while bakers were able to turn out more loaves of bread due to the faster baking techniques, the nutritional value of the bread was lost.

Among those that Metcalfe and Graham influenced was Amos Bronson Alcott, father of *Little Women* author Louisa May Alcott. A writer, philosopher, and educator, Alcott was a proponent of transcendentalism, which began as a reform movement within the Unitarian Church and proposed that the soul of each individual is identical with the soul of the world and contains what the world contains. In 1843, he and educational reformer Charles Lane established Fruitlands, an ambitious utopian community in Massachusetts. Gathering together a small but eager group of disaffected intellectuals, Alcott advocated an austere vegan lifestyle, stating, "The entrance to paradise is still through the straight and narrow gate of self-denial. Eden's avenue is yet guarded by the fiery-armed cherubim, and humility and charity are the credentials for admission." The diet at Fruitland consisted of fruit, grains, beans, and peas. All animal flesh and by-products were forbidden due to their corrupting nature, and tea, coffee, rice, molasses, and sugar were off-limits because they were produced by slave labor. The community's goal was to produce only what they needed; they believed that the acquisition of material goods inhibits spirituality. For a time, Alcott admired the self-supporting activities of the Shaker community but ultimately condemned them for indulging in production and trade with the outside world. As well-intentioned as Fruitland's goals were, successful communal living required more than a well-tended vegetable garden and discussions of philosophy; Alcott's experiment lasted just seven months. Louisa May Alcott wrote of her experience at Fruitland in *Transcendental Wild Oats;* Fruitland stands today as a museum.

Adventists and Cornflakes and Vegans—Oh My!

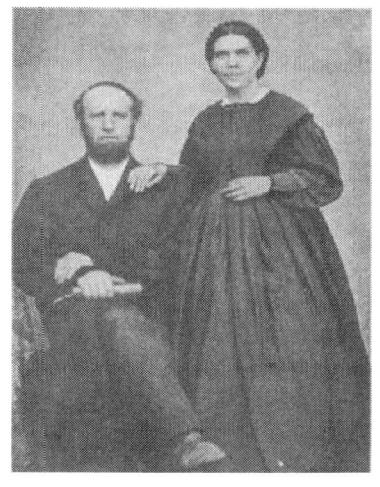

The Seventh-day Adventist (SDA) Church, founded in the 1840s by vegetarian health reformer Ellen White, was one of biggest influences on modern-day vegetarianism in the United States. Ellen believed that the proper diet for humans was prescribed by God in the Bible, and wrote in 1864 that Adam and Eve were given all they needed for nourishment: "He designed that the race should eat. It was contrary to His plan to have the life of any creature taken. There was to be no death in Eden. The fruit of the trees in the garden was the food man's wants required." The SDA Church focuses heavily on spiritual health, diet, and exercise; in fact, several studies have found that Adventists are significantly healthier than the general population. Today, almost all of the church's clergy and roughly half of its two million members worldwide are ovo-lacto-vegetarians, and the SDA Church owns a publishing company and a number of hospitals, natural food stores, and vegetarian restaurants. Church-affiliated universities are leaders in scientific research into dietetics and continue to promote vegetarianism with a strong emphasis on health.

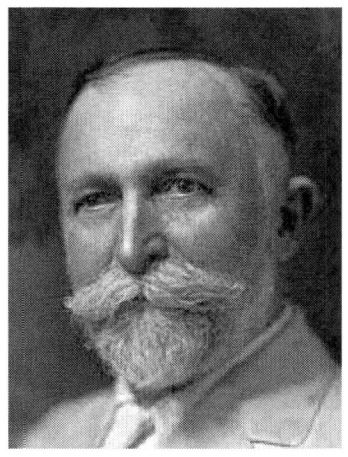

John Harvey Kellogg was a man who worked as a printer for White and helped publish the Adventists' health journal. White and her husband, James, took a liking to Kellogg, paid for his medical school education, and! then placed him in charge of their Battle Creek Sanitarium— a spa retreat for health restoration and training. A believer in the value of preventative medicine, Dr. Kellogg's treatments were founded in the Adventist philosophy with an emphasis on fresh air, sunshine, exercise, rest, and diet. The diet he prescribed and which he called "biologic living," forbade the consumption of meats, condiments, spices, alcohol, chocolate, coffee, and tea, but he worked tirelessly to create a vegetarian diet that was also varied and tasty. Over the course of his career, Dr. Kellogg invented over eighty different products using nuts and grains; these included peanut butter, a cereal-based coffee substitute (an early version of Postum), and cornflakes.

Dr. Kellogg was convinced that many illnesses were caused by toxic bacteria in the bowels. He favored a high-fiber vegetarian diet, blaming some 90 percent of all diseases on stomach and bowel problems. He was especially concerned about the effects of a nonvegetarian lifestyle on the intestinal tract. In many ways, Dr. Kellogg's practices can be viewed as downright goofy. He disapproved of sexual activity of all kinds, gave patients multiple daily enemas, and administered shock therapy in electrified tanks of water, but his influence as an advocate of vegetarianism was profound. Among the visitors to his sanitarium were automobile tycoon Henry Ford, retailers J.C. Penney and S.S. Kresge, actress Sarah Berhardt, explorer Richard Byrd, inventor Thomas Edison, industrialist Harvey Firestone, President William Howard Taft, and aviator Amelia Earhart. Once he started marketing his food products, Dr. Kellogg had to hire his brother to take over because the enterprise was so successful. Numerous competitors copied his method of mass production of cereal for the marketplace.

Battle Creek Sanitarium was just one of many vegetarian health retreats in the United States, and advocates of the lifestyle—and shrewd businessmen hoping to capitalize on a trend—opened vegetarian restaurants in large cities across the country. Toward the end of the century, however, interest in vegetarianism waned. In the early part of the twentieth century, the United States Department of Agriculture (USDA) began producing food guides ostensibly to help struggling families plan nutritious meals during inflation and food rationing. These food guides, unsurprisingly, recommended that Americans eat hefty amounts of meat, eggs, and dairy—all products of the food industries overseen by the Department of Agriculture.

The Swingin' '60s: Peace, Free Love, and Vegetarianism

Vegetarianism regained some popularity in the 1960s with the teaching of Michio Kushi, an advocate of macrobiotics who founded the Kushi Institute in Massachusetts. Born in Japan, Kushi came to the 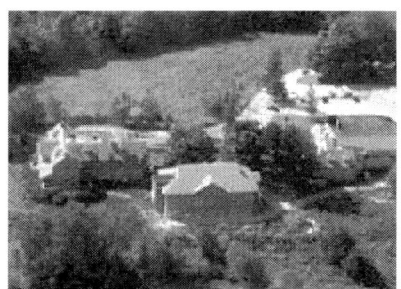 United States in 1949, eager to share what he'd learned from macrobiotic educator Georges Ohsawa, who taught that food was the key to health and that health was the key to peace. In Boston, Kushi founded Erewhon, the country's pioneer natural foods distributor, making organically grown whole foods and naturally processed foods widely available and introducing countless people to miso, tofu, tempeh, sea vegetables, barley, malt, rice syrup, azuki beans, and rice cakes. The mainstream availability of health foods that we have today simply wouldn't be possible if it was not for Michio Kushi. Throughout the 1980s, Kushi met government leaders at the United Nations and around the world, promoting macrobiotics and working hard to convey the philosophy of healthful, thoughtful eating.

But the real vegetarian boom came in the early 1970s following the publication of Frances Moore Lappé's *Diet for a Small Planet*. Published at a time when the world was beginning to register alarm over depletion of the earth's resources, Lappé's book raised awareness about the wasteful manner in which animals were reared for consumption as meat. Though not a vegetarian herself, Lappé promoted eating in healthful, respectful ways that made a gentler impact on the environment. Her book advocated a complicated methodology for eating complete proteins that involved combining food low in certain amino acids with other foods high in that amino acids. In later editions of the book, she abandoned that method, saying, "In combating the myth that meat is the only way to get high quality protein, I reinforced another myth. I gave the impression that in order to get enough protein without meat, considerable care was needed in choosing foods. Actually, it is much easier than I thought." While Lappé's book was slow to gain popularity, in the three decades since its release, it has sold over three million copies and spawned a 2002 sequel, *Hope's Edge: The Next Diet for a Small Planet,* in which Lappé once again looks at the way we feed ourselves. In 2001, Lappé and her daughter, Anna, founded the Small Planet Institute, a research and educational organization which partners with foundations, individuals, and socially responsible businesses to promote "living democracy," a philosophy of sustainable and positive working communities.

The ethical side of vegetarianism also received a boost in the mid-1970s with the publication of the book, *Animal Liberation,* by ethicist Peter Singer; it argued against what the author called "speciesism" or discrimination based on the belief that humans own animals and can do whatever they like with them. He believed that the use of animals for food was unjustifiable because it created unnecessary suffering. His contention that all beings capable of suffering should be granted equal consideration helped to promote not just vegetarianism but a vegan lifestyle. A few years later in 1975, the nonprofit group People for the Ethical Treatment of Animals (PETA) was formed, founded on the tenet that "animals are not ours to eat, wear, experiment on, or use for entertainment." In addition to high-profile campaigns against animal testing and fur farming, PETA has lobbied passionately against the use of animals for food. The group has had great success in uncovering and stopping inhumane treatment of animals in laboratories and in spreading awareness of veganism, particularly through their Lettuce Ladies—lovely young women dressed only in bikinis made from lettuce—and a 2003 advertising campaign which compared animals killed in factory farms with concentration camp victims.

So Where Are We Now?

Vegetarianism is now more popular and acceptable by mainstream society than ever before. With growing cases of diabetes, heart disease, and cancer, and the rise of meat-borne illnesses like E. Coli and Mad Cow disease, a vegetarian diet is a smarter option today than at any time in the past. In a world where our natural resources are being depleted at a rate far faster than they can possibly be renewed, it makes more sense than ever to walk gently on the planet. Fortunately, the ranks of vegetarians are swelling as people figure these things out for themselves. With any luck, most of the world will come around to the vegetarian way of thinking while we still have some of its resources left.

CHAPTER 3

Ethical Eating
Why Becoming a Vegetarian is Good for You and for the Earth

Some people become vegetarians because they simply find meat unappetizing—chewing and digesting chunks of animal flesh isn't their idea of fine dining. And that's a perfectly valid reason to embrace a vegetarian lifestyle. But for many others, vegetarianism is part of their commitment to living their lives with as much environmental, moral, and political responsibility as possible—and becoming a vegetarian is a natural part of that resolve.

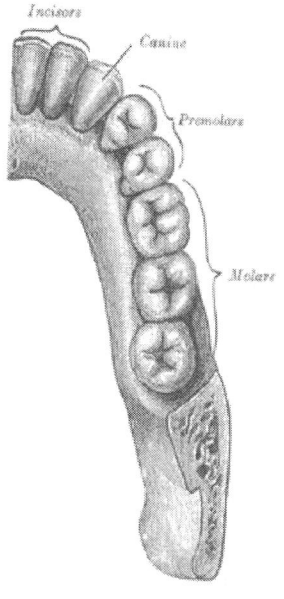

In fact, just because humans can digest meat and metabolize the protein, that doesn't mean we were designed to eat meat as a primary nutritional source. Yes, we *can* eat meat, but the way our bodies are built shows that we function more efficiently on plant foods. One clue is the design of our teeth. If you examine the teeth of true carnivorous animals, theirs are long, sharp, and pointed in the front for the purpose of tearing away flesh. Our so-called canine teeth—the four teeth in the front corners of our mouths—are very poorly designed for the task when you compare them to the teeth of dogs, cats, lions, and wolves. Human teeth are short, blunt, and only very slightly rounded on top—not designed to tear at meat at all! Similarly, the lower jaws of meat-eating animals open very wide but move very little from side to side, and this adds power and stability to their bite. Like other plant-eating animals, our jaws not only open and close but also move forward, backward, and side to side; they are designed to bite off pieces of plant matter which are then grinded into smaller pieces by the flat molars.

But the most important evolutionary development that sets humans apart from other animals is our huge, overdeveloped brain. We have the ability to choose what we eat and how we live; we aren't just eating machines forced by the circumstances of nature to eat a specific diet. As a human, you can make decisions based on science, ethics, morals, and good old-fashioned common sense.

Every choice you make has repercussions, from the excess packaging that you toss in the trash (plastic and cardboard that ends up in a landfill) to the light bulbs that you use (most likely manufactured by a company that supplies nuclear triggers to bomb manufacturers). The food you choose to eat is no exception. In our industrialized Western world, meat appears in tidy wrapped packages in our grocer's shop, so we don't usually think about where it came from—the resources used to raise the animal, the additives pumped into the feed to increase production, and the manner in which the animals live and die. But every time you buy meat, you support the system that created it, and chances are, you have no idea just what that entails!

What's the Beef with the Cattle Industry?

One of the most eye-opening revelations in Frances Moore Lappé's provocative 1971 book, *Diet for a Small Planet,* was the information on the environmentally disastrous impact of the beef industry. According to Moore, one of the biggest effects was on the groundwater supply that we used for drinking, cooking, and bathing. In the United States alone, the various underground water tables are dropping from six inches to six feet per year. Today, even as our water supplies are dwindling, almost half of the water in the United States each year is used to irrigate land to grow food—with vast quantities of that going to produce the grain that's fed to farm animals.

The rate of return—the amount of food we get for the amount of water we use—on animal protein is pretty poor. As an example, it takes about twenty-three gallons of water to produce a pound of tomatoes. Compare that to the estimated at least two thousand gallons of water used to produce a pound of beef. In her book, Lappé called cattle a "protein factory in reverse," meaning they consume more protein than they provide! For every pound of beef that a steer provides, it eats seven pounds of grain and soy protein. So, from the environmental point of view, doesn't it make more sense to just eat the grains?

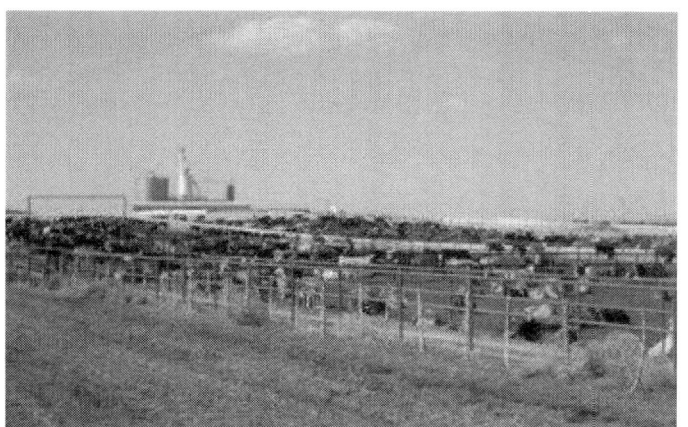

As global warming due to air pollution becomes an even more dire development, scientists are looking not only to the pollutants produced by cars and factories, but to that produced by factory farming as well. Cattle produce methane gas (and if you've ever driven past a stockyard, you know how dense that gas can be!), and methane makes up 9 percent of the gases contributing to the greenhouse effect—approximately seventy to eighty tons of methane per year. They also produce waste high in nitrous oxide, another factor in global warming. In fact, animal waste is the largest source of nitrous oxide emission in the environment, making up 95 percent. As more and more rain forest is leveled to create pastures for grazing, cattle farming in these cleared areas also contributes to global warming. And the runoff from cattle farms—containing nitrogen, phosphorous, waste-borne pathogens, and detergents—often flows directly into the waterways, destroying fish habitats and leaching into the groundwater that is used for our daily needs.

Then there's the massive use of fossil fuels required to get beef to the market. Today's massive, high-tech factory farms burn fuel to run the machinery that provides heating, lighting, and cooling, in addition to the gasoline that fuels the trucks that deliver the feed and transport the cattle and meat to the market. The Worldwatch Institute estimates that it takes about forty-eight gallons of gasoline to provide the red meat and poultry that an average American consumes in a year.

Old McDonald Doesn't Live Here Anymore

Ah, the pastoral pleasures of farm life! Fluffy sheep grazing contentedly in the fields, the chickens clucking in the henhouse, and the pigs happily munching away on the family's leftovers from their communal trough. Everyone's happy and healthy and doing their part for the cycle of life.

Unfortunately, real-life farms are not at all like that. At least, not in this day and age of mass-quantity factory farms where the well-being of animals is hardly considered and the only issue is how to harvest as much meat for market as is possible per square foot of land. To that end, farmers now forgo traditional grazing practices and pack as many animals as possible into crowded feedlots, where they do nothing throughout their short lives but eat tons of grain and drink thousands of gallons of water. Dairy cows are often treated better than beef cattle, but increasingly, dairy farmers are keeping their cows housed inside barns, where they develop leg and hoof problems due to standing continuously on cement floors. Cows today are also forced to produce more milk than ever before; they are constantly milked by machines with little rest, causing them to develop painfully inflamed udders. The forced milk production shortens their lives too. When treated well, cows can live for up to twenty years, producing milk for over half their life. Today's dairy cows are so overmilked that they can only produce for three or four years, after which time they're sent to the slaughterhouse.

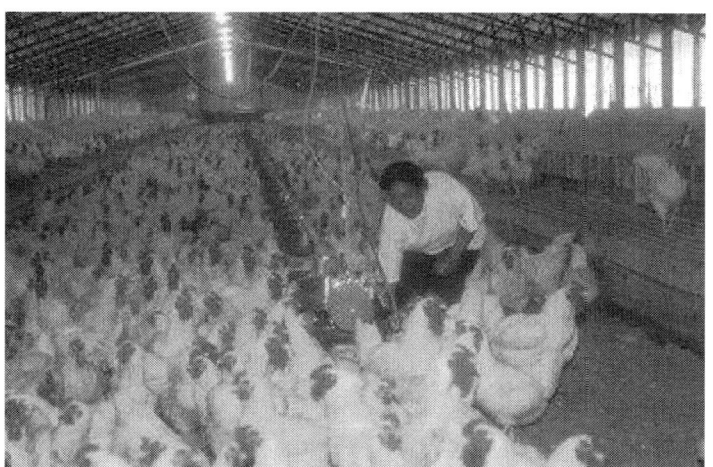

Cows aren't the only animals to suffer under factory farming practices. Chickens are treated especially poorly, living their entire lives in cramped confinement. They are crowded so closely together that they're debeaked— their beaks are snapped off with a machine tool—so that they don't harm each other with their hysterical pecking. Debeaked chickens have difficulty eating, which isn't surprising, and live in such terrible conditions that they're forced to eat their own and other chickens' feces along with their food; this contributes to the wide variety of potentially deadly bacteria that gets passed onto the consumer.

Besides the debeaking, another unpleasant practice is molting. Chickens produce more eggs when they shed their feathers, so egg farmers induce the egg-laying state by starving the birds for up to twelve days at a time. Besides being inhumane, some researchers have concluded that forced molting increases chickens' levels of salmonella. This also assists egg farmers in weeding out the weaker hens—about 3 percent of chickens die of starvation during the forced molting process. In fact, the entire egg-production process starts with killing. Male chicks have no function on a modern egg farm and are culled by workers whose job consists of identifying them and tossing them, while still alive, into machines that grind them up and add them to the hens' feed. Practices like this, along with molting and debeaking, have caused such a public outcry that even the McDonald's Corporation couldn't ignore it. In 2000, the fast-food giant sent letters to the farmers who provided the over 1.5 billion eggs that they use each year, demanding that chickens be housed in larger cages and that forced molting be stopped.

Campylobacter

The most frequently contaminated of all meat in the United States is undoubtedly chicken. The poultry industry is the first to admit that a lot of the chicken they sell contains Campylobacter bacteria. Most of you have probably never even heard of Campylobacter bacteria, because it is not reported on nearly as much as E. coli. But, in reality, this specific kind of bacteria kills more Americans every year than E. coli, and the death toll continues to rise. The bacteria get into the mucosal layer of the intestines and cause a disease that can be recognized by bloody diarrhea, fever, body aches and pains, and abdominal discomfort. Unlike other food poisoning, symptoms don't usually arise until a week after ingestion. *The Food Revolution* reports that 40 percent of the cases of the Guillain-Barre syndrome, a life-threatening condition of paralysis, often followed the onset of an infection from Campylobacter bacteria. Although the poultry industry is well aware of the threat of Campylobacter and what causes it (contaminated litter or the bedding of the chicken coupe), they refuse to do anything about it because of the extra financial cost.

How This Little Piggy Gets to Market

Pigs are friendly and gregarious and are counted among the most intelligent of the domesticated beasts. Those who raise pigs—the ones who care about their animals—say that they're as smart and as loving as dogs or cats; they enjoy music, bask in the sun, and play with toys. They're also very clean animals that only wallow in mud to cool off and keep away flies. All of this makes it especially horrifying when you learn how they're treated in factory farms.

Mother pigs on farms in the United States live out most of their lives in gestation crates that are only six feet in length and two feet wide—too small for them to even turn around. They display signs of boredom and stress when confined in such a

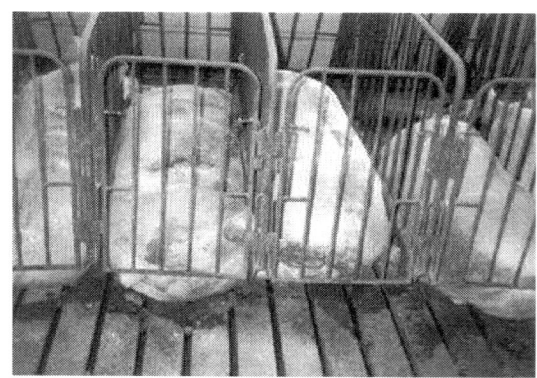

manner, biting the bars of the cage and gnashing their teeth. Piglets' tails are often routinely cut off so they won't bite each other on it, a neurotic behavior that only occurs in confinement. Piglets are taken away from their mothers three weeks after birth, then packed into pens until they are singled out to be raised for breeding or for meat. Often, the piglets' teeth are chipped off with pliers to further discourage them from biting each other.

For transport, pigs are stuffed into trucks with no food or water and without any temperature regulation. During the midwestern winters, they often freeze on the sides of the trucks or die from dehydration. According to numbers provided by the pork industry, over a hundred thousand pigs die on their way to slaughterhouses each year, and over four hundred thousand arrive crippled due to barbaric transport practices. At the slaughterhouse, the pigs are stunned with an electrical charge to their brain or heart which, when done correctly, immediately renders them unconscious before they're tossed into tanks of scalding water which softens their skin and removes their hair. However, stunning is often done incorrectly—meaning that the pigs are still conscious and already in severe pain when they're thrown into the scalding water. Audits of factory farms by the USDA and independent organizations continually find scores of slaughter rule violations. One PETA investigation uncovered a plant in Oklahoma where workers killed pigs by slamming their heads against the floor and beating them with hammers.

Fish Have Feelings Too

Some vegetarians think that eating fish is a suitable alternative because they believe that fish aren't subjected to the torture that cattle and pigs experience. This isn't the case. As an effort to help curb the world hunger crisis, fish farming or aquaculture has become quite popular. Several researchers have found that, as a direct result of aquaculture, some populations of herring, mackerel, sardines, and other fish low in the marine food chain are in danger of disappearing altogether from the world's oceans. Just like cattle, chickens, and pigs, raising large numbers of fish in a closed, unnatural environment puts an unusual amount of stress on the fish, which increases possibility of outbreaks of disease both on the farm and in the surrounding waters. This in its turn has led to an increase in the use of chemicals and antibiotics to control the outbreaks.

Fish are also poorly treated on fish farms. As many as forty thousand fish are kept in one small cage with barely enough water to survive. Fish in the wild can swim thousands of miles during the duration of their life. Caged fish can hardly move. Most consumers are not aware that the fish they are eating come from fish farms. In 1990, about 6 percent of the salmon consumed in the world were the product of fish farms. By 1998, the number was 40 percent. Ten years later, the number is even higher. Unfortunately, many people make the false assumption that farmed fish is more environmentally benign. Yet, aquaculture causes enormous waste problems. For example, caged salmon farmed in Scotland contaminate coastal waters with waste that is produced by a whopping eight million people. Other repercussions of fish farming, in addition to coastal pollution, include the destruction of natural landscapes and forests, and the displacement of people living in those areas. In 2000, a report by the *New Internationalist* stated that the environmental damage caused by fish farming could be compared to that of replacing tropical rain forests with cattle ranches. Unfortunately, the fish farming industry has basically followed in the footsteps of the cattle, poultry, and pork industry.

To sum up, if you are becoming a vegetarian based on practical, moral, or ethical reasons, consider cutting fish out of your diet as well as beef, poultry, and pork. There are viable alternatives that are healthier for all.

Vegetarianism—The Thoughtful Alternative

There are many, many benefits that you'll see immediately when you become a vegetarian, including clear skin, shiny hair, and lower risk of high cholesterol, diabetes, and kidney disease. But the wider benefit is the one you can't see: the benefit to the rest of the world. Keep the following facts in mind when you feel tempted to go back to eating meat.

You're helping to conserve water. Water is the earth's most precious resource, and currently about 50 percent of the water in the United States is used to grow crops for grain-fed animals—as opposed to 35 percent that's used to grow food crops for humans to eat. It takes roughly 15 times as much water to produce the same amount of protein from an animal that we can get from plant sources. By 2025, two-thirds of the world will face shortage of water. This will most likely lead to difficulty in food production, overpopulation in certain areas, and civil unrest. Switching to a vegetarian diet is the single biggest thing that you can do to cut down on your consumption of water.

You're helping to protect the land. Livestock grazing erodes topsoil, drying out the land and making it unusable for farming. This is one reason why forests are being cut at an alarming rate to make room for more cattle grazing. Agriculture accounts for nearly 90 percent of the thirty million acres of rain forest that are destroyed each year. Nearly 25 percent of all prescription drugs have a basis in rain forest plants; destroying the rain forest may mean destroying our chances of curing cancer or AIDS.

You're helping to conserve fossil fuels. In this supply-and-demand world, less demand means less production, which means less consumption of fossil fuels. Animal agriculture uses more than a third of the fossil fuels consumed in the United States; a calorie of animal protein requires ten times as much fuel as is needed to produce a calorie of plant protein. Researchers at the University of Chicago compared the amount of fossil fuel needed to cultivate and process various foods and the amount of fuel that's used to operate agricultural machinery, provide food for livestock, and irrigate crops. They also factored in emissions of methane and nitrous oxide produced by cows, sheep, and manure treatment. According to the findings, the average American diet that consists of about 28 percent animal foods generates an equivalent of 1.5 tons more carbon dioxide each year than a comparable vegan diet. The researchers pointed out that driving a hybrid car rather than an average vehicle would conserve a little over one ton of carbon dioxide per year—meaning that living a vegan lifestyle reduces more emissions than is done by driving a hybrid car!

You're making a more compassionate choice. Now that you've read about the horrors of factory farming, do you think that slice of bacon really worth it? There's a famous quote from George Bernard Shaw: "When a man wants to murder a tiger he calls it sport; when the tiger wants to murder him he calls it ferocity." Many people believe that we have a natural right to kill and eat animals, but imagine a time when an alien species visits our planet. They're smarter than we are, have technology far more advanced than our own, and they like to eat meat. So humans become the factory-farmed animals taken to slaughterhouses; as we cry and scream and fight to no avail, we're shoved into pens until such time as we're marched onto the killing floor, bashed in the head, and stripped of our flesh, which is then neatly packaged for market. It's a horrible thought, yet that's what humans do to animals every day. St. Francis of Assisi said, "If you have men who will exclude any of god's creatures from the shelter of compassion and pity, you will have men who will deal likewise with their fellow men." Choosing a vegetarian lifestyle is choosing the path of compassion.

How We Treat the Food We Eat

Farming has been a part of human history, but the old way of farming in which the animals' best interests were at heart is long gone. The people who raised animals for meat, milk, eggs, and more took care of their flock or herd. They knew that if any of the animals fell sick, their entire farming operation would be at risk. Farmers had a vested interest in making sure their animals were properly cared for. They placed animals in an environment that was conducive to their way of life, such as grazing areas for cows and sheep. But the twentieth century brought industrialization and, with it, industrial farming.

Farming factories began sprouting up everywhere. Animals are now kept in overcrowded factories where hormones and other antibiotics are used to keep them healthy (though many of them still die prematurely because of the restricted environment). You probably don't think about the way animals are treated when you sit down to eat a nonvegetarian meal. But that's normal. Most people don't stop and think about the food that they eat. Why would they? They don't have a clue about how animals are raised and processed because a lot of the information isn't being passed along to the consumer. If the truth about the way animals were treated was more accessible, there'd be more vegetarians than meat eaters in the world!

Feeding the World with Plants

Considering the vast resources squandered to provide consumers with meat, it's obvious that it's an illogical and inefficient way to feed our continually growing population. Vegetarian diets can sustain far more people than diets that revolve around meat. When we eat grains, vegetables, fruits, nuts, and seeds, we're eating the food that is fed to the meat animals that are later, in turn, eaten by us. It just doesn't make sense. Factor in the damage to the earth, the water, and the air ... on a global level; our reliance on animal foods is devastating.

There's some debate as to whether your choosing a vegetarian diet really helps to feed other people. There simply isn't enough food to feed the world, but that's an issue combined with far more complicated problems of politics, distribution of food, and geography than just choice of diet. But one thing is certain: Westerners eat way more food than they need. In poorer nations, the average person eats about a pound of grain each day. In the United States, it's four times that amount, and a large part of that is the grain used to produce the animal proteins we eat. While people are starving all over the globe, the United States feeds 70 percent of its harvested grain to animals—meaning that most of the food we grow goes to produce even more food that much of the rest of the world can't afford to purchase.

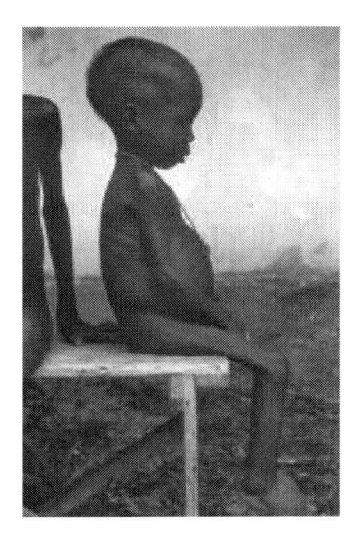

The increase of nonvegetarians around the world is directly contributing to hunger and will continue to do so unless something drastic is done. Worldwide, meat production quadrupled from forty-four million tons in 1950 to 195 million tons in 1996. Countries like China and India—both with a long, rich tradition of vegetable-based diets—are becoming increasingly avid consumers of meat. In China alone, pork consumption has risen astronomically in the last decade; the Chinese now consume more pork per person than an average American. And while India still has the largest vegetarian population in the world, the country is now also the largest exporter of meat in Asia. There just isn't enough grain to support these industries, much less feed people directly. In 1993, China exported eight million tons of grain, but thanks to its expanding pork industry, the country imported sixteen million tons of grain just two years later in 1995. Eating meat is almost universally seen as a symbol of economic progress, but the more meat humans eat, the more humans there are that go hungry.

If more people embraced vegetarianism, it's highly likely that far less animals would be fed and killed for meat. A widespread conversion to plant-based diets would reduce food shortage simply by reducing the number of factory-farmed animals and their drain on land and other resources. With fewer animals to feed, it might be possible to rebuild world grain reserves and guarantee that there's enough food for even the poorest countries. And reducing the amount of worldwide animal agriculture would contribute to biological diversity, climate control, and restoration of the ozone layer.

World hunger is an issue too huge to comprehend. Ultimately, though, your conscience is your guide. Knowing what you now know, do you still feel good about eating a hamburger? Albert Einstein said it best: "Nothing will benefit human health and increase the chances for survival of life on Earth as much as the evolution to a vegetarian diet." By choosing a vegetarian lifestyle, you're choosing to be a caring citizen of the world.

In addition to the explanations listed above, here are ten good reasons why you should become a vegetarian.

1. Vegetarian diets are healthy and low in fat.

2. Vegetarian diets actually contain a good amount of protein.

3. Vegetarian diets are responsible and compassionate.

4. Meat is unhealthy for you and the earth.

5. Vegetarians care about the environment.

6. Vegetarian diets can help reduce world hunger.

7. Vegetarians help conserve water.

8. Vegetarian diets help preserve land and forests.

9. Vegetarian diets help eliminate the use of fossil fuels.

10. Vegetarian diets can lead to longevity.

CHAPTER 4

Where Do I Begin?
Getting Started on Your Meatless Journey

If you've made it this far, you're obviously ready to change your life and become a vegetarian. But giving up meat—especially if you've become accustomed to making it your main source of protein—can be challenging. You'll find, as you go along, that it involves more things than just changing the foods that you eat. You're going to have to adjust the way you think about nutrition, your body, your self-image, and how your choices affect the world you live in. But it's also a deeply personal voyage that's yours to undertake in your own way; it will involve finding the path that will take you into the future in the healthiest and happiest way possible.

It may not be an easy transition either. You may still love the taste of meat, and the idea of living your entire life without it would be daunting. You may have family members who are resistant to making the change and who will try to sabotage it for their own reasons. You'll need to learn new recipes, plan new menus, and arm yourself with nutritional information that you never bothered with before. It's a lot to think about!

It can all seem overwhelming, but with a plan, some structure, and a little guidance, it can be done by anyone. The most important thing is to be patient. Allow yourself the time you need to develop new menus that you enjoy, try new recipes, and discover new foods. Don't think that becoming a vegetarian means that you'll be spending countless hours wandering the aisles of natural food stores and figuring out what to do with quinoa—unless you enjoy that sort of thing. The truth is, the easiest way to transition to a vegetarian diet is to eat foods easily available at your neighborhood grocery store—although you'll definitely want to check out that health food store as you become more comfortable with your vegetarian lifestyle.

Finding a Sense of Purpose

To successfully switch over from a lifelong habit like eating meat to the healthier habit of living entirely on plant-based foods, you'll need a strong reason for changing. If you aren't 100 percent sure of your reasons for becoming vegetarian, you'll find it hard to resist temptation. Social pressure is often the undoing of new vegetarians—they're completely committed when at home or eating out with another vegetarian, but they give in to meat cravings when presented with a friend's meat loaf or attending an outdoor barbecue. I was the same way until I found a way of thinking that helped me to stick with the vegetarian lifestyle.

When I first started to become a vegetarian, I fell off the wagon many times. I'd be a committed vegetarian for days, then give in to some form of temptation (I still craved for KFC!), feel bad about myself, then try again. And again. I kept improving all the time, eventually sticking to my vegetarian diet for weeks at a stretch. I stayed true to my new lifestyle for three months, and then a friend took me to a seafood buffet, and I gave into temptation yet again! I wanted to become a vegetarian because I hated the idea of killing animals for food, but sometimes those foods were very hard to resist.

I earnestly wanted to become a vegetarian, yet I kept failing. Why? How could I want to do this so much and still fail? After a lot of soul searching, I found my reason to be a real vegetarian, and I haven't looked back since. Once I knew, with every part of my mind and heart, why vegetarianism was so important to me, I was able to commit to it completely and to discard all desire to eat meat again!

Here's the reason that I found works for me. Like most people, I don't want to be hurt, killed, or to receive pain, and animals certainly don't want those things either. They feel pain, just like we do. So isn't it wrong to inflict pain and death on animals? Just because humans have better technology, we often believe that we're superior to other living beings and that we can do whatever we want to them. This isn't the case. All living things are connected. What we do to animals, we do to ourselves.

In an earlier chapter, we discussed the concept of an alien race coming to earth and believing that they were superior to humans. We would be nothing to them—much the same way as we look at cows, pigs, and chickens—so they would very likely think, "These humans are a low, primitive species. We can do whatever we want to them since they can't fight back. We have complete control over them." If these aliens were not vegetarians, there would be nothing to stop them from herding us into pens, cutting off our feet and hands so that we couldn't run or fight back, kill us in slaughterhouses, and then eat us for food. Let's be honest; we taste great! So, they would kill millions of us every day, cut us up into steaks and chops, store the meat, and sell it to each other in little white, plastic-wrapped packages.

It's a horrible, horrible thought. Yet this is exactly the way we treat animals right now, because we believe we are superior to them and we have better technology. But is this really the right way to treat other living beings? Animals feel happiness and fear, pleasure and pain. They just want to live, which is their purpose for being.

Think about that. They just want to live. Who doesn't want to live? What right does humanity have to decide the time and the manner in which an animal's life should end?

That's my personal reasoning for becoming a vegetarian. Once I came to the realization that harming and killing animals for my food was wrong and completely unnecessary, I was no longer tempted by meat. I found my reason to stay committed. My journey with meat has ended. And I've been a vegetarian ever since. You need to find your own reason that can strike such a strong chord with you intellectually and emotionally that you will never have to look back at your previous life—a reason that you believe so strongly, you'll never regret the decision, because you know that it's the right thing to do.

If you found my reasoning persuasive, go ahead and use it as your own. Whatever reasoning you choose, make it something that you believe in with your whole heart. Once you do, vegetarianism will be something that you can adopt completely for your entire life.

Look on the Bright Side!

The best way to make stress-free changes in your eating habits is to keep your mind on the benefits of your new diet. Many nonvegetarians think that vegetarians must have a painfully boring diet and eat only brown rice, broccoli, and other vegetables. But in truth, most vegetarians have much more adventurous and interesting diets than your average Mr. Meat-And-Potatoes. Crack open a few vegetarian cookbooks, and you'll find delicious recipes drawing from cuisines with long histories of vegetarian eating—foods loaded with spices and exotic flavors from India, China, and the Mediterranean. Add those to the vegetarian foods you already love—like macaroni and cheese, vegetable soup, pasta with marinara sauce—and you'll find there's a whole world of delicious things you can enjoy!

How long it takes for you to fully embrace vegetarianism is entirely up to you. Some people give up meat in one fell swoop, deciding in an instant that, for moral, ethical, or health reasons, the time to give up meat is now, and they never look back. Other people transition slowly, giving up meat-based foods one meal at a time over a long period. Many take the "two steps forward, one step back" approach, falling off the meatless wagon here and there on the road to a plant-based diet. None of these methods is the right way; the right way for you will be the way that works! And there are methods that can make the change easier.

A radical dietary change can take a lot of getting used to, both mentally and physically. And while a vegetarian diet is absolutely the best, healthiest way of life, not everyone can dive straight into the deep end right away. Many people take a long time to slowly make the changes necessary to live a vegetarian lifestyle—and transitioning gradually is often the most enjoyable, low-stress way to do it.

Before we outline a ten-point plan for gradually transitioning to a vegetarian diet, let's take a look at the pros and cons of making a quick change versus making a gradual one.

Tearing Off the Band-Aid—Making the Quick Transition

There are a number of benefits to making a one-step switch to meatless eating. They are:

You can feel good about changing your life right away. There's something deeply gratifying about taking decisive action and making positive changes in your life. You reach your goal right away, and you get to say to yourself, "Yes. I'm a vegetarian!"

You'll enjoy the benefits of vegetarianism starting on the very first day. By making a major life-altering change right away, you'll see the results much sooner. This is especially important if you're going vegetarian for health reasons such as losing weight or lowering your cholesterol.

There's less concern that you'll fail and never become a "total" vegetarian. For some people, doing things gradually just isn't an option—they lose focus and never make it to their goal. If you're the sort of person who has a history of giving up on diets before you've reached your target weight, or on hobbies before you master the craft, you may want to make the change in one big jump. There's nothing wrong with the decision; you just need to own up to it and act accordingly.

The quick approach works best for people who've already educated themselves on basic vegetarian nutrition, have a strong support system in place (living or working with vegetarians, or having a partner who's also making the change at the same time), and don't have other stressful situations while trying it. Again, only you can determine if this is best for you. Many people find the gradual approach just doesn't work for them because they lose their motivation during a slow dietary overhaul, but others do much better at making huge changes slowly over a long period of time.

You may choose to make a quick change to vegetarianism because you have no other choice. You may have seen a documentary on factory-farming practices and just can't stand to eat meat again. You may have been diagnosed with a condition like diverticulitis—which causes small pockets in the intestine to harbor bacteria—and your doctor may have advised you to stop eating meat. If that's the case, you won't be able to do your homework ahead of time, but you can still do the best you can with the information in this book and other resources that you'll discover as you go along.

There are, of course, a few drawbacks to this method. You'll be changing a major part of your everyday life without any learned skills and without the education that comes with experience. You'll be springing your new vegetarian lifestyle on your family, friends, and co-workers all of a sudden, and you will have to deal with their reactions. If you're bombarded by negative feedback from those around you, you may find that your new way of eating is kicked to the curb before it really starts.

But, as mentioned above, many people thrive on this kind of change. You may find that giving up so many of your old habits all at once helps you to break unhealthy old patterns and seek out new recipes and menus right from the start. If that's the case, keep an eye out for bumps in the road, look for support—whether from other vegetarians you know or on the Internet—and check out the chapters in this book dedicated to nutrition and meal planning.

Easing In—The Gradual Approach to Going Meatless

Taking changes one simple step at a time makes the process more manageable and, for many people, makes the entire transition seem far less daunting. It also makes it fun—with each step, you change a little something, learn some new information, and try a few things you've never tried before! As you master each new skill, you become more confident in your ability to maintain your new lifestyle, plan your meals, and handle yourself in any number of social situations.

There are two main advantages to taking a gradual approach to switching to vegetarianism. They are:

You're more likely to make the changes permanent if you change your habits slowly. By changing your habits gradually, you change the way you think about eating as you go along; you learn more and create a strong base on which to anchor your new, better, healthier habits.

Making a number of small changes gives you the chance to adapt them to your current lifestyle as you go along. You probably have so many things in your everyday life going on at once that you often feel overwhelmed already. Making a slow transition is simply less disruptive to your life than making one huge, sweeping change.

The downside to the gradual approach, as we've already discussed, is that you might find yourself losing focus and taking longer to complete the transition to a completely vegetarian lifestyle. If you take too long, you will never make it to your goal. Be honest with yourself. If it's been months since you started changing habits and you're still not there, you may want to take a hard look at where you are, where you want to be, and what steps you need to take to get there.

There is also a possibility that if you make changes slowly, you may get stuck in one place and stay in a state of semivegetarianism permanently. You might decide to stop eating red meat but never move on to giving up fish and chicken. You might intend to eventually eat an entirely vegan diet, yet you never give up eggs and cheese, and end up feeling like a failure. So if you want to make a slow transition, plot out the changes you intend to make, set specific goals, and follow a structured plan.

What to Do When the Going Gets Tough

Once you've made the transition to vegetarianism, the importance of maintaining your meat-free resolve is ever-present. As with any new way of thinking and/or living, you have to expect a couple of bumps in the road or a few hiccups along the way to vegetarianism. But don't get frustrated with yourself. Use the adjustment period as a time of experimentation. Try new recipes and new foods at home. When you go to a restaurant, sample new vegetarian dishes. Read up on nutrition, and let yourself adjust properly to a vegetarian-driven mindset.

Giving up meat for the rest of your life can seem like a daunting task. As with anything you eat in moderation, you're going to get cravings. That is why you should reduce your meat intake slowly (review the Ten-Point Plan to Becoming a Vegetarian). Occasional slipups are completely normal. Don't be too hard on yourself. Change takes time and patience. Always remember to take it one step at a time. When you are in a situation where you don't have the option to stick to your vegetarian diet, just pick up where you left off the very next day.

A lot of people tend to look on the bright side of life. Others ... not so much. Focusing on the restrictions of a vegetarian diet instead of the benefits can cause a lack of focus and will make maintaining discipline that much harder. It's all about the way you choose to look at your plate. Instead of focusing on the meat that isn't there, focus on all of the nutritional goodness that is there. Any vegetarian will tell you that they have more foods to choose from than most people think. The varieties of vegetarian meals are endless. And a positive attitude can make all the difference in the world. More choices mean more meal options and more plates full of yummy food. Don't waste precious time and energy thinking about what you used to eat. Think about what you haven't even tried yet. Get excited about planning your meals and tasting new vegetarian dishes. Eventually, you'll forget all about the missing meat, and maintaining discipline will become second nature.

Add a little fun to the vegetarian transition process by keeping a record of the foods you used to eat and the ones you eat now. Track your progress down on paper, and watch your diet evolve right before your eyes. Jot down thoughts about cravings and why you crave those foods. In time, you may notice an unhealthy pattern build around certain foods. Having a sense of awareness about the food that you choose to eat will help you step outside of the box and see things on a much larger scale. You may realize that you were craving meat or other foods not because you liked the taste of them but because you were conditioned to eat them. Writing is a healthy form of expression and can certainly help you in your transition. Take pride in how far you progress, study the before and after mindset, and take notes on the vegetarian foods you like and dislike. All of this will help keep you focused on the task in hand and serve as a crutch when you are having an off day.

Your Ten-Point Plan to Becoming a Vegetarian

For those craving guidance and structure, what follows is a simple ten-step transition from a nonvegetarian to a veggie lifestyle. Of course, you don't have to follow this course of action to become a vegetarian, but sometimes having a carefully thought-out plan in place before beginning a major venture can make you feel more secure about the unfamiliar path you've chosen to take. You'll notice that, at the beginning, it is only making changes to your evening meals. Dinner is perhaps the single most planned meal of the day; it is the meal that the family eats together, putting thought into planning the main course, side courses, and dessert.

If you think about the variety in your current diet, you'll discover that you already draw from only a handful of recipes to make family favorites over and over again and rely on basic meals that you enjoy and have made before. You may go out to a new restaurant for a special occasion or try a new recipe now and then, but we all keep going back to tried-and-tested favorites several times a month. Planning vegetarian meals is no different. During the steps of your transition, you'll discover a number of delicious new meals, revise current favorites to make them vegetarian, and have as many meal options at your disposal as you did as a meat eater—maybe more!

As you develop healthy new habits and learn more about nutrition, you'll find that your previous ideas of what constitutes a complete evening meal will change drastically. Ever since the era of *Ozzie and Harriet,* we've been told that an appropriate family dinner includes a large portion of meat, some veggies on the side, a starch of some sort, and, often, a big glass of milk. Soon you'll be abandoning that idea; eating a healthy satisfying vegetarian diet isn't just a matter of replacing meat with something else while continuing the same old method of consuming four squares. A quickly put together veggie stir-fry with a multigrain roll is a fast, nutritious evening dinner—so is homemade macaroni and cheese accompanied by a green salad. The old ways of eating don't apply to you anymore, so go ahead and forget what you were taught about meal planning; you're about to develop your own rules based on what your body needs.

Step 1: Eat three meat-free dinners during the week that you already enjoy.

Make a list of vegetarian main dishes that you and your family already like—macaroni and cheese, vegetable soup with bread and salad, cheese quesadillas, vegetable stir-fry, and quiche and cheese pizza are just a few of the meatless meals you already eat. This still leaves four nights a week that you can include meat in your meals, but you've taken the first step toward thinking differently about your eating habits.

Step 2: Adapt three favorite recipes to make them vegetarian, and add them to your week's dinners.

A wide variety of main course meals can be turned into delicious vegetarian fare, allowing you to enjoy healthier versions of foods you already love. Take a recipe for vegetarian chili and make it your own by using the same mixture of spices in your own ground beef chili; leave the beef out of your lasagna, and replace it with sautéed zucchini, eggplant, and mushrooms; make your favorite soups and stews using coarsely chopped portabella mushrooms; mix up a zesty taco salad with the usual lettuce, tomatoes, sour cream, and salsa, but replace the ground beef with a mixture of black and kidney beans. The possibilities are only as limited as your imagination!

Step 3: Add three brand-new vegetarian meals to your repertoire.

During the previous two steps, you developed six vegetarian dinners that you and your family are happy to eat. Now it's time to do a little research and find a few new tricks to spice up your menus even further with some new recipes. Purchase a couple of vegetarian cookbooks, borrow them from friends, or check them out in the library. We'll provide you with some great recipes in chapter 13 to get you started.

You can also search the Internet for recipes; online vegetarian support groups are a terrific source of recipes from veggie lovers. Find recipes that look tasty, and give them a try. This is a time for experimenting; if something doesn't appeal to you after you've served it up, discard that recipe and try something else. No matter what your level of cooking expertise is, there are recipes you can make, and you'll even find yourself becoming a better cook as you develop new skills.

Step 4: Make all your dinners meatless.

Once you've found three new dishes that you love for dinner, that's nine vegetarian dinners to choose from! If you like, you can have a different meal every night, plus two alternates—which may be more variety than you had before you started transitioning to a meatless diet! Odds are that, at this point, you'll be intrigued by the different flavors and textures of your vegetarian entrees and that you'll keep on creating new menus.

After all, you're not going to eat the same nine things for the rest of your life—but it's a great way to start! With so many dinners to choose from, it's time to ban meat from your dinner table entirely. You should feel secure that you're not going to go hungry with so many options and that you will discover even more in future.

Step 5: Give up the lunch meat.

Now that you've successfully given up eating meat during your evening meal, it's time to turn your attention to your lunches. If you're the sort of person who visits a restaurant to take a lunch break from office, look for places that offer vegetarian pasta options, vegetarian (or vegetarian-friendly) cafes, and places that have well-stocked salad bars. Burger places probably won't have much for you to eat, but spots that specialize in sandwiches usually have vegetarian options. The downtown areas of many big cities also have street vendors offering Indian, Thai, and Mexican vegan specialties.

If you eat at home or take your lunch to work, you'll naturally have a lot more control over your meal planning. If you have a microwave at work, you can heat up a bean burrito, a frozen vegetarian meal, or leftovers from your evening meals. A snackish meal of pita bread slices, hummus, and fruit is nutritious and fun, and if you're ovo-lacto, there's always egg salad or grilled cheese.

Step 6: Change your old breakfast habits.

Breakfast doesn't have to be eggs, bacon, and sausage. It can be anything you want it to be! If you want cheese enchiladas or leftover vegetarian chili, go for it. A fruit smoothie with a scoop of alternative protein powder is a quick breakfast that'll give you the boost you need, or you can toast a couple of pieces of whole-grain bread and top it with peanut butter.

On weekends, when you have more time to cook and linger over breakfast, make an omelet stuffed with mushrooms, onions, and cheese, or a stack of blueberry pancakes. If you simply can't shake the craving for breakfast meats, there are vegetarian sausage links— including even fake bacon made from vegetables that are great for you— which can help satisfy the craving. Just remember that breakfast is whatever you want it to be; so long as you're getting the nutrition you need, you can eat anything you like.

Step 7: Get creative.

If you've gotten this far, it's time to get serious about embracing the vegetarian lifestyle. Giving up meat is only the beginning; there's a whole world of foods to explore, ranging from grains, seeds, and nuts to vegetables you've never tried before. The more foods you're open to eating, the more creativity you can bring to your cooking. At this point, you should be feeling pretty good about the meal choices you already have under your belt, so now is the time to start having fun and trying new things.

As you thumb through vegetarian cookbooks, you'll find recipes that use exotic ingredients like quinoa, tahini, and spelt. Try using rice milk as a replacement for cow's milk in recipes, and experiment with exotic spice combinations that you've never tried before. This is your chance to develop a broader, more interesting recipe repertoire. Enjoy yourself! You can also take a trip to your local health food co-op store and spend awhile reading the labels on all the products you've never seen before. Don't be intimidated by the unfamiliar labels and ingredients, and don't be shy about asking the employees for tips on how to use foods you find intriguing, or for recommendations and recipes. Tell them up front that you're new to vegetarianism, and they'll be happy to point you toward foods you've probably never considered before.

Step 8: Giving up the eggs.

During the last step, you may have noticed that you're now an ovo-lacto-vegetarian! Congratulations! You may also notice, though, that you're eating a lot of eggs and cheese. This happens to most new vegetarians, because cheese is tasty and eggs are an inexpensive source of protein.

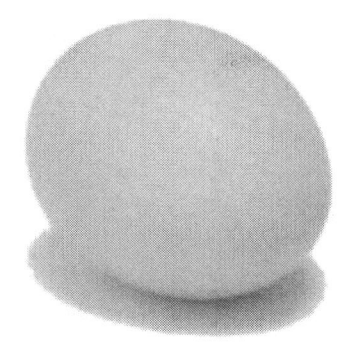

But both cheese and eggs add fat and cholesterol to your diet, and, if you think back to previous chapters, the practices of high-tech egg farms are barbaric. Experienced vegetarians know how to replace eggs in recipes, and now that you're an experienced vegetarian too, it's time you started doing the same. You certainly don't have to give up eggs entirely if you don't want to, but there are a number of ways that you can at least cut back on the amount of eggs you eat. If you're a fan of egg salad, try replacing the eggs with chickpeas; use everything else you would in your favorite egg salad recipe, like mayonnaise, celery, onion, and mustard, and you'll find that you never miss the eggs. Chickpeas also work as an excellent substitute for scrambled eggs when sautéed with onions, mushrooms, garlic, and a little salt.

When making a veggie loaf or vegetarian burger, try some tahini (chickpea paste available in the natural foods or ethic section of your grocery store) or mashed potatoes as a binding agent. After some experimentation, you may find that you don't want to give up eggs after all. But even then, cutting back on your consumption is a good idea for a number of reasons, and you can always seek out organic eggs from small, local farms that don't indulge in the same abhorrent practices as the big ones.

Step 9: Find new ways to build your bones.

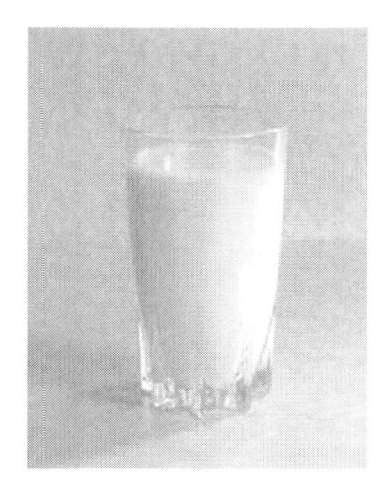

When we're kids, we're all told over and over again to drink our milk. Even as adults, the milk industry keeps drumming into our heads that we have to drink milk and eat lots of dairy products to maintain strong bones and teeth. While it's true that our bodies require calcium for good health, we don't need to drink milk to get it. Did you know that humans are the only animals who drink the milk of other species? Cow's milk is ingeniously designed by nature to provide the calcium, riboflavin, fat, protein, and carbohydrates that a baby calf needs—and even calves stop drinking milk once it is past infancy.

Humans have actually evolved over thousands of years in a way so that many of us—mostly Westerners—can drink milk without getting sick; our intestines produce lactase, an enzyme that breaks down the sugars (lactose) in cow milk. But many non-Western cultures have never developed the ability to drink milk, and a large number of people of European descent are still lactose intolerant. Drinking milk as an adult is simply unnatural—people who can do so without suffering intestinal discomfort are benefiting from a genetic anomaly.

Yet, we still need calcium. If you enjoy eating cereal, try one of the many hemp milk or rice-based milk replacements on the market. There are a wide variety of brands and they all taste different—so if you don't like the first one or two you try, keep experimenting until you find one you like. And make sure you add calcium-rich food to your meals like leafy green vegetables and beans. We'll discuss this is further detail in the next chapter.

Once you find yourself enjoying a wide variety of foods that are rich in calcium, you'll find it a lot easier to eliminate dairy from your diet. After you become accustomed to eating calcium-rich foods and drinking nondairy milk supplements, you can move on to trying soy-free cheeses. And look for nutritional yeast at your health food store; added to dishes or sprinkled on popcorn, it adds a delicious, cheeselike flavor to recipes.

Step 10: Become a savvy consumer.

When you shop for food, examine the labels carefully for animal products you need to avoid. You'll be surprised by how many foods contain lard, dried milk, eggs, and other animal by-products. It can be extremely challenging at first, but don't be discouraged. You'll soon find yourself becoming as familiar with the products and brand names that help you stay on course as you were with the products you used in your old lifestyle.

As you spend more and more time educating yourself about being vegetarian, you'll discover exactly how diligent you want to be about your new lifestyle. You may find that it's worth the effort you put into it, and you may want to embrace a completely vegan way of life. Or you may find you are comfortable eating commercially made bread products that contain eggs while not cooking with eggs for your other meals. Don't allow politics to dictate your dietary choices, seeing a vegan diet as ethically superior to an ovo-lacto one, and beating yourself up because you still eat cheese. You can be proud of yourself for adopting a vegetarian lifestyle, and even if you don't go 100 percent vegan, you've still made a healthy, humane choice. Congratulate yourself!

CHAPTER 5

Vegetarian Nutrition

Getting Everything Your Body Needs

At this point you're probably starting to get worried about how you're going to make sure you get the right balance of nutrients that your body needs and thinking that you'll need a spreadsheet to keep track of everything you eat. But it's not as difficult as it may seem from the outset; you just need to hone up on a few nutritional basics to keep in mind when you plan your meals.

Some people spend their entire lives studying the science of nutrition, but you don't have to make it your life's work. The truth is, despite what the meat industry repeatedly tells you, vegetarian diets aren't nutritionally inferior to nonvegetarian ones. There's no need to worry that you'll be lacking the vitamins, minerals, and protein that your body needs—which isn't to say that it's not possible to eat badly as a vegetarian; many people have lousy diets, even vegetarians. But if you eat smart, your vegetarian diet can be the healthiest way you've ever eaten.

Protein—Am I getting enough?

Your first concern on starting a vegetarian way of life is that, without meat foods in your diet, you'll lack protein. So you'll be happy to discover that it's almost impossible to eat too little protein on a vegetarian diet.

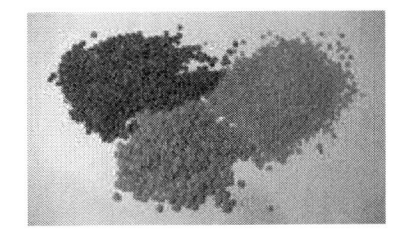

Protein is of utmost importance to a healthful diet. Your bones, muscles, and hormones all contain protein, and eating enough of it helps keep your body strong on the most fundamental level. Unfortunately, eating animal protein for the purpose has long been made unrealistically important. Man once believed that eating the flesh of other animals would make him stronger and healthier, but now that we know the dangers of eating saturated fats, it's obvious that limiting animal proteins is the healthy choice.

Vegetarians can, of course, be protein deficient, but that is caused by undereating or relying too heavily on junk foods. In most cases, any diet adequate in calories from a variety of healthful sources provides enough protein. Grains, vegetables, beans, seeds, and nuts are all protein-rich foods and easily provide all the nutrition the body needs.

Contrary to what many vegetarians believed in the last couple of decades, you don't need to weigh and balance arcane combinations of foods to get adequate protein. This myth goes back to Frances Moore Lappé's 1971 book, *Diet for a Small Planet*, in which she wrote that vegetarians needed to balance foods based on which amino acids they were lacking by creating complementing proteins. For some time, there were even nutritionists who created complex charts to help vegetarians pick foods that went together, and concerned vegetarians made sure to combine beans and rice, rice and corn, or grains and cheese—it was an awful lot to remember!

We now know that combining types of protein isn't nearly as important as simply consuming enough calories to maintain a healthy weight. Lappé even revised later editions of her book, admitting that she was wrong about the importance of food combining. If you eat enough food from different sources, you'll probably be getting plenty of protein.

If you want to get technical about it, health professionals recommend that you eat 0.8 grams of protein each day for every kilogram of body weight. A kilogram is about 2.2 pounds, so to find your recommended amount of daily protein, multiply your ideal weight by 0.8, and then divide that number by 2.2. If you prefer a quicker method, just divide your ideal weight by 3. But even then, you don't need to eat that much protein to stay healthy. Keep in mind that recommendations like these always err on the side of safety, so the number you get will actually be higher than what you realistically need. I would advise you not to get too technical; remember that there are people who have gone vegetarian for several generations and they all lived healthily without problems. In fact, most vegetarians never count the amount of protein and other vitamins they consume each day, just like nonvegetarians.

But you, as a vegetarian, should strive to meet the recommended daily requirement of protein because plant proteins are, unfortunately, less efficient foods for providing nutrients. For one thing, ovo-lacto-vegetarians consume a similar amount of protein to omnivores, and vegans who eat a lot of wheat grains also get plenty of protein.

It'll always be true, however, that as a vegetarian you're eating less protein than people who eat both plant and animal proteins. A 1984 study found that a typical omnivore diet consists of 15 to 17 percent protein, while lacto-ovo-vegetarians generally eat about 13 percent protein and vegans around 11 to 12 percent. Despite needing more protein and eating less, the vegans still had an adequate amount of protein in the diets. So don't worry about doing anything fancy to meet your protein requirements. Just eat from a variety of sources and get enough calories and you'll be fine—you will, in fact, be better than fine because nonvegetarians generally eat too much protein!

Studies have shown that replacing animal protein with plant protein in your diet can help lower your blood cholesterol levels and reduce your risk of heart attack. Most people are by now aware of the danger of saturated fats in red meat and its effect on blood cholesterol. People recovering from heart attacks are prescribed diets which replace the beef with skinless chicken or fish. That is a good move, to be sure, but these people could lower their cholesterol even further by switching to a vegetarian diet and reducing the amount of fat that they eat. Plant proteins are free of cholesterol and lower in saturated fat than animal proteins and dairy products.

There are also studies that show that eating slightly less protein than is optimal is far better than eating too much, and in this era of supersizing, most nonvegetarians eat far more than they need. When we eat too much protein, our kidneys are responsible for filtering out the excess. In the process, calcium is lost, increasing the risk of osteoporosis. Since plant-based diets are lower in total protein, vegetarian diets are better for your bones! Excess protein is also, understandably, hard on the kidneys and unhealthy for people with kidney disease.

Plant proteins contain all the same amino acids, to differing degrees, as animal proteins, and eating enough of them gives you all the protein you need. Studies have shown that people can meet their protein needs just by eating rice, wheat, or potatoes so long as they meet their caloric needs. By eating a variety of plant foods throughout the day and consuming enough calories, you'll be getting enough healthy plant protein. You'll have a lower risk of heart and kidney disease, and you'll be eating protein that's more efficiently produced using less valuable resources than animal protein. It's what people call a "win-win situation!"

Quick Tips for Finding the Right Protein Balance:

> 1. Aim for 0.8 grams of protein for every kilogram of your body weight.
>
> 2. Find out which foods are rich in protein and whether or not you eat these foods on a regular basis already.
>
> 3. Remember that too much protein results in a buildup of calcium.
>
> 4. Understand that vegetarian daily diets already contain enough protein.
>
> 5. As long as you are getting enough calories to meet your energy needs, it's practically impossible to lack a decent amount of protein

Protein-packed Foods:

> Bean burritos
> Oatmeal
> Cereal and hemp milk

Veggie burgers
Red beans and rice
Black beans
Vegetarian chili
Vegetable soup
Lentil soup
Falafel
Pasta with marinara or pesto
Black bean burgers

Building Bones with Calcium

Calcium is vital to avoid bone-threatening diseases like osteoporosis, yet in countries where people eat the highest amount of calcium and protein, the highest number of hip fractures, a symptom of osteoporosis, have been recorded. Scientists are coming to the conclusion that there's more to osteoporosis than just the amount of calcium we eat; overall lifestyle plays a large part, including physical activity levels and environmental factors. Just eating four to five servings of calcium-rich foods each day is no guarantee that you'll avoid osteoporosis, but it'll certainly be a step in the right direction.

Dairy industry propaganda tells us that milk does the body good, but that's simply not true. Over two-thirds of the people in the world are lactose intolerant and find it difficult to digest milk. The cause is an insufficient amount of lactase, the enzyme that breaks down the sugars in milk, in their metabolic system. Undigested, the mucous lactose coats the lining of the colon, bacteria interact with it to cause gas, and the result is cramps, flatulence, and diarrhea. All mammals are born with a sufficient amount of lactase, but it decreases as we get older. Once we're out of infancy, we're not meant to be drinking milk any longer.

But while we don't need to drink milk, we still need calcium. Almost all of the calcium in our bodies at any given time is stored in our bones and teeth, with about 1 percent in our bloodstream. And that's the calcium that's the key to good health; it's needed to send messages between nerves, especially those that contract our muscles. It's also a vital component in the clotting of blood. Our kidneys filter most of our bodies' calcium and return it to the bloodstream, but some of it is lost in our urine. We also lose some through sweat and bowel movements.

Our bones are constantly breaking down (don't worry—they build back up) replenishing calcium into our blood. Somewhere around the age of thirty, our bones stop growing and reach maximum density. This is why calcium is most important when you're young; the denser your bones are when they reach this stage of development, the less is the chance of your getting osteoporosis when you're older. That's because after the age of forty-five, our bones break down faster than they're rebuilt; at this point, we start to lose as much as 0.5 percent of our bone mass each year. So by the time we hit sixty-five, bone loss can start to be a real problem. Women lose even more bone mass when they reach menopause, as they stop producing estrogen, the hormone that protects our bones.

We can't increase the density of our bones once they stop growing, but we can slow the rate at which calcium disappears from our bones by making sure that we eat calcium-rich foods. This holds true whether you eat an omnivorous diet, an ovo-lacto diet, or a completely vegan diet—there is no firm evidence that vegetarians have stronger bones than people who eat meat or weaker bones either. But some nutritionists believe that vegetarians may actually need less calcium to keep their bones strong.

How can that be? Well, protein from plant sources are metabolized by the body in different ways than animal proteins. Meat contains more sulfur-containing amino acids than plant proteins, which makes the blood more acidic. To neutralize the acid, your body needs more calcium—and what it doesn't find in the bloodstream it pulls from our bones. That calcium then leaves your body through your urine, taking even more calcium from your kidneys along the way.

In addition, sodium takes a heavy toll on your body's calcium supplies, and along with table salt, sodium is added to canned foods, cured meats, soft drinks, condiments, and snack foods. When you think of the amount of protein and sodium your average American consumes during a day full of bacon cheeseburgers, ham sandwiches, sodas, and French fries, it's not hard to see why they need more compensatory calcium than does your average vegetarian!

So how much calcium do you actually need? Well, a good rule of thumb is to eat between two and five servings of calcium-rich foods—

leafy green vegetables, broccoli, beans, and, yes, dairy products are among your choices—while keeping your protein and sodium intake moderate. The recommended calcium-to-protein ratio is 16:1, so if you want to calculate your calcium needs, you'll need to estimate your protein consumption first.

Surprisingly, even bread can be a good source of calcium. It was once thought that fiber and phytates, substances found in grains and nuts, bind to calcium and the human the body lacked the mechanism to absorb it. However, when yeast is present, it breaks the bond between phytates and calcium, allowing it to be used by the body, so yeast-raised breads, especially whole-grain breads, can provide a substantial amount of calcium. Also, some leafy greens are less effective sources of calcium than others—Swiss chard, spinach, beet greens, and rhubarb contain substances called oxalates, which limit the absorption of calcium (but they're still chock-full of iron, so eat them anyway).

Eating a variety of foods every day makes for a more interesting, enjoyable vegetarian way of life, so it makes sense to get your calcium from many different foods. Adequate calcium is especially important for growing children (we'll address vegetarian kids in chapter 17) so they build the strong bones they'll need when they're older. But you don't need to get your calcium from milk. As we've discussed here, milk isn't even good for you! Plant foods like leafy green vegetables, rice products, fortified orange juice, and dried beans are loaded with calcium. And they make your menus much more fun!

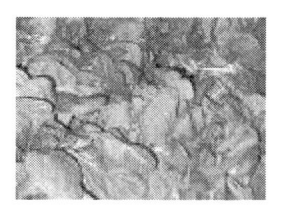

Our Friends, the Vitamins

There are thirteen vitamins that have been determined as necessary to human health. They're divided into two classes: water-soluble vitamins, the excess of which is excreted through urine or through sweat; and fat-soluble vitamins, the excess of which is stored in our bodies. Vitamin C and eight B vitamins are water soluble, so if you take too much of these, your body just gets rid of what it doesn't need. Vitamins B12, A, D, K, and E are fat-soluble; any excess of these are kept in our bodies for some time, and we can overdose on them if we take too much.

Fat-soluble vitamins are so called because they need dietary fat to be absorbed by the body. A diet exceedingly low in fat makes it difficult for the body to use these vitamins, although it's only a small amount of fat—vitamin absorption is only an issue in the most extreme cases. They're needed for a diverse array of bodily functions, from blood clotting to eyesight to the immune system. Water-soluble vitamins already exist in the body's enzyme system and are necessary to keep the body functioning smoothly. A handful of these vitamins are especially important to the vegetarian diet, and it's crucial that you know why you need them.

Vitamin B12—The Everything Vitamin

One of the most controversial nutritional elements is vitamin B12, of which you need only the tiniest amount—just two micrograms per day. One tiny pinch would be enough for you to meet your body's needs for your whole life. So how small an amount do you actually need? Look at it this way: one microgram is one thirty-millionth of an ounce.

B12 is created by microorganisms that exist in the air, water, and soil. Animals, including humans, have it in their bodies. We consume vitamin B12 by eating the flesh of animals that pass it along, or by consuming animal products like eggs, milk, cheese, and yogurt. Vitamin B12 is also produced in our own intestinal tracts, but scientists believe that produce it past the point where we can absorb it into our blood streams—so we can't utilize the B1 we produce ourselves. We have to get it from somewhere else.

Plants only contain B12 through contact with them, passed on through the soil. So if you eat vegetables straight from the garden, you may pick up a little bit of B12 from soil present on the plant. But if you buy all your veggies from the grocery store, they'll have been cleaned well enough to remove the tiniest speck of B12. So where the heck do we get B12?

Coming as it does from minuscule bacteria, there are a number of forms of vitamin B12. The one that we humans need and that our bodies can use, is called cyanocobalamin. Other types of B12—the types we can't utilize—are called analogs. For years, nutritionists lectured that B12 was abundant in foods like nutritional yeast, tempeh, and sea vegetables. But it turns out that, while there's lots of B12 in those foods, it's mostly of the type we can't use, despite the claims on the labels. Up to 94 percent of the vitamin B12 in those foods is in analog form and not cyanocobalamin, so these foods are essentially worthless as sources of B12.

There are some vegetarian food choices that contain a decent amount of vitamin B12. Breakfast cereals like Wheat Chex or Grape-Nuts, meat substitutes such as Morningstar products, milk substitutes, eggs, and most dairy products all provide a good amount of B12. If you don't eat animal products on a regular basis, then you need to find an alternate source.

One foolproof way to add B12 to your diet is through fortified food products and vitamin supplements. Read labels carefully, and look for the word "cyanocobalamin"; you should be able to find plenty of breakfast cereals and meat substitutes fortified with the right kind of B12. If you decide to go with a vitamin supplement, choose one with the lowest dose available. Remember, you only need two micrograms a day, and most supplements contain much more than that. The reason to keep your daily dosage low is because your body actually adapts to the amount of B12 you get from supplements and your diet; it's going to absorb just what it needs and discard the rest. So why take a big dose when you'll only absorb two micrograms?

Also keep in mind that you really only need a B12 supplement if you're eating a vegan or near-vegan diet. If you're ovo-lacto, you'll get all the B12 you need from the foods you eat.

Riboflavin, Your Little Yellow Friend

If you've ever taken a megavitamin and have been alarmed later at the bright yellow color of your urine, you've met vitamin B2, also known as riboflavin. Like all of the B vitamins, riboflavin plays a part in the complex enzyme reactions that make everything in your system work. Nutritional scientists believe that vitamin B2 plays a part in more of the body's various functions than any other vitamin, so when you don't get enough, it can cause a number of disparate dysfunctions like anemia, skin problems, a swollen tongue, dry cracks at the corners of the mouth, or neurological problems.

Riboflavin is naturally present, in small amounts, in a number of foods, and the amount you need is directly connected to your energy intake; the more calories you need, the more riboflavin you require. The recommended daily requirement of riboflavin is 1.7 milligrams per day for men and 1.3 for women, but many experts now believe that the numbers are high—many people eat far less than the RDA of riboflavin and never show any signs of deficiency.

A number of plant foods contain moderate amounts of riboflavin, so it is easy to get the amount you need from the foods you eat. Leafy greens, broccoli, yogurt, legumes, and avocados are sources of riboflavin, and enriched breads and cereals are good sources as well. You can make sure that your vitamin supplement contains vitamin B2 but, as with so many nutrients, simply eating a healthy diet that includes a variety of foods will ensure that you're getting enough.

Vitamin D, the Sunshine Vitamin

Vitamin D is of course a vitamin, but it also falls under the same general classification as hormones; our body generates it for use by another part of the body later. We create vitamin D through exposure to the sun, then it goes to our bones, kidney, and intestines to regulate calcium and strengthen our bones. Hundreds of years ago, people suffered regularly from diseases like rickets and osteomalacia due to inadequate exposure to sunlight. Thankfully, such cases are rarely seen today.

To generate enough vitamin D from the sun to help your body all year round, you need about half an hour's exposure to sunlight on the hands and face three times a week with no sunscreen. If you have darker sun, you'll need more exposure. Lighter skin, however, will require less. However much you need, the exposure you get during the summer and spring is supposed to carry you through the long winter. It's possible to not get enough vitamin D, especially if you live in an area that has a heavy smog layer, spend all of your days indoors, or regularly go outside wearing heavy clothes and sunscreen. Older people are at a greater risk of vitamin D deficiency, as our ability to manufacture it decreases with age.

The good news is that if your vegetarian diet includes dairy, you're probably getting enough. In the United States, dairy products are fortified with vitamin D, and extra supplements aren't necessary. Vegans (and others who forgo dairy products) may want to take supplemental vitamin D. If so, you may want to consult with a nutritionist or other health professional—excess vitamin D gets stored in the body, creating calcium deposits that can damage the kidneys and heart.

The best solution? Get outside in the sun!

Don't Underestimate the Importance of Iron

Much like protein and calcium, most people associate iron with meat products. They assume that the only source of iron is red meat. Actually, iron is quite prevalent in plant products. Iron is extremely important to the body because it helps carry oxygen in the blood to the cells of the body. It also helps provide oxygen to the muscles for energy. When you do not have enough iron in your body, you will most likely feel lethargic.

Despite popular belief, vegetarians are not prone to anemia or iron deficiency. The recommended daily allowance of iron varies depending on your gender and age. The recommendations for women are generally higher because women tend to lose more iron through menstruation. Although vegetarians may need more iron because the iron in plant-based products is not easily absorbed, you'll be surprised to know that, on average, vegetarians normally consume more iron in their diets than nonvegetarians. Vegans tend to get more iron than vegetarians because they do not eat dairy products, which tend to contain very little iron.

All you have to do to get the required amount of iron in your vegetarian diet is to be aware as to which foods contain the most iron and to eat plenty of fruits and vegetables that are rich in vitamin C (vitamin C is one of the most powerful iron-absorption agents).

It's easy to find iron in everyday foods if you just take a look around.

Iron-rich foods include

      Breads and cereals
      Legumes
      Nuts and seeds
      Fruits

Vegetables
Blackstrap molasses (a couple of teaspoons is all you need)

The basic premise of iron absorption has to do more with absorbing agents than it does with the actual consumption of iron. Meat is a great source of iron because it is an iron-absorption enhancer. Of course, vegetarians don't eat meat. Thankfully, there are foods that vegetarians can eat which also serve as iron-absorption enhancers.

Iron-absorption enhancers

Broccoli
Brussels sprouts
Cabbage
Cantaloupe
Cauliflower
Citrus Fruits
Green and Red Bell Peppers
Honeydew
Kiwi
Strawberries
Papaya
Potatoes
Tomatoes

Now we know that there are iron-absorption enhancers available. But did you know that there are iron-inhibitors as well? There are some substances in the food we eat that actually inhibit your body's natural ability to absorb iron. Certain spices, calcium in dairy products, and the caffeine in coffee all decrease your body's ability to absorb iron. Tea is the worse iron-inhibitor, so if you drink a lot of tea, be especially aware of your iron intake. You might even consider switching to herbal tea because herbal tea does not contain tannic acid, which is an iron-inhibiting agent. Your body's ability to absorb iron also depends on the degree in which you need iron in the first place. If you are slightly anemic, your body may not be getting enough iron-absorption enhancing foods. But, the human body is a natural wonder. It adapts to all situations and will only absorb as much iron as it needs. It's important to make sure you are getting enough iron in your diet but, as with anything else, always remember that there is such a thing as excess.

The Rest of the Best

Vitamin B1 (thiamin) helps convert carbohydrates to energy, and we need about 0.5 milligrams for every 1,000 calories we eat to do the job. The disease beriberi, famous from countless jungle adventure movies, is caused by a deficiency of thiamine and results in damage to the nervous system. Vegetarians generally get lots of thiamine in their diets; whole grains are loaded with it, enriched breads offer a lot of B1, and nutritional yeast is a good source too.

Vitamin B6 (pyridoxine) is a component of sixty different enzyme systems, most of which help your body metabolize protein; the amount you need is based on how much protein you eat. Vegetarians, who consume less protein overall than omnivores, need less B6. Since plant foods contain very high levels of B6 for the amount of protein they offer, vegetarians usually get plenty of B6. There's even more good news for vegetarians. Studies have shown that animal proteins actually increase the need for B6 more than plant proteins, so people on meatless diets need about 25 percent less. It's also been found that the type of B vitamins offered by plant foods is less susceptible to destruction during cooking than those in meat, so vegetarians win there too.

Folic acid, also called "follate," is necessary for metabolization of protein and for efficient cell division in the body. It works with B12 to create new material needed for the cells to divide and grow. The current RDA is 200 micrograms for men and 180 micrograms for women. Vegetables are great sources of folic acid, especially broccoli, leafy greens, and asparagus. Legumes also contain a lot of folic acid, so eat your black-eyed peas.

Vitamin C was once believed to cure colds, but we now know that the best you can hope for is that large doses will reduce the severity of a cold. Lack of vitamin C also causes scurvy, once the scourge of seafaring folk who lacked fresh vegetables on long voyages. Odds are, you're not a pirate or a merchant seaman, so you probably don't need to worry about your intake of C as it's abundant in fruits and vegetables, especially citrus fruits, strawberries, peppers, watermelon, potatoes—yes, potatoes!—and broccoli. Vegetarians get more than the recommended amounts from the foods they eat, and vegans get the most vitamin C of all!

CHAPTER 6

Parasites

The Guests Who Came to Dinner

The intestinal tract is like a luxury hotel for parasites, bacteria, and fungi. It's warm, it's moist, and oxygen is limited due to all the waste matter that's packed in there. The colon—one of the most important organs in the body—is a dumping ground for waste, the place where the body toxins and excess nutrients that could be harmful to the system go. It's also where your body absorbs the nutrients that it needs in order to function and survive—so the health of your colon is mighty important. Parasites in particular can be dangerous to the health of the colon, leeching nutrients from the body and emitting harmful toxins that can further weaken the colon's integrity. This can lead to a number of problems, from the mildly annoying to the deadly, such as:

- Blood sugar imbalances
- Bloating
- Sugar cravings
- Fatigue
- Insomnia
- Weight gain or loss
- Teeth grinding or TMJ
- Diarrhea
- Itching
- Irritability
- Malnutrition
- Anemia
- Immune deficiency

It's estimated that over 90 percent of Americans contract a parasite of some kind at some point in their life. They enter our bodies from a variety of sources, including pets, food, and unwashed hands. You can pick up parasites from contact with pets and other people or just by walking barefoot on the street. Children are easily infected because they are less aware of hygiene and play with dirt and other possibly contaminated substances. But meat consumption is probably the biggest contributor to parasites flourishing in our bodies.

Eating meat can cause constipation, and constipation creates the perfect environment for parasites to thrive. These unwelcome guests multiply in the *haustras*, the pouches in the colon where debris is stored. At their least offensive, they cause intestinal gas—but if you experience any of the symptoms above, even something as seemingly minor as chronically itchy skin, you could very well be harboring parasites in your colon.

There are several families of parasites: roundworms, tapeworms, flukes and single-cell parasites. Each group has its own unique subset of parasites that do different things to your body. Let's look at some of the more common intestinal parasites and what you can do to avoid them.

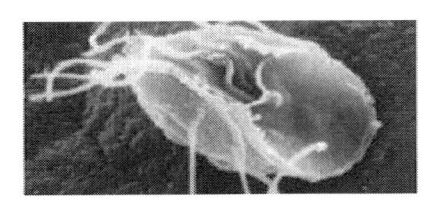

Giardia lamblia are protozoan parasites that infect humans via consumption of contaminated food and water. They are commonly found in untreated water supplies and are one of the most common causes of diarrhea in travelers, but people sometimes pick them up while swimming in ponds and lakes. Giardia is responsible for the condition known as giardiasis that causes diarrhea, bloating, flatulence, abdominal cramping, weight loss, greasy stools, and dehydration.

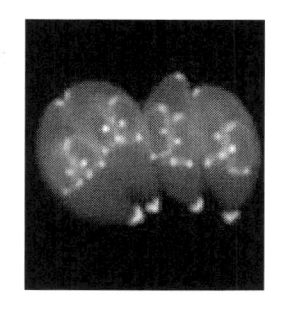

Toxoplasma gondii is another protozoan organism commonly found in the colon. Cats and kittens often carry it, and it can be transmitted to humans who handle cats, and particularly their feces. You can also be infected with them by breathing in their eggs. Toxoplasma is responsible for the disease *toxoplasmosis,* which causes chills, fever, headaches, and fatigue. If a pregnant woman contracts toxoplasmosis, it can lead to miscarriage or birth defects such as blindness and mental retardation.

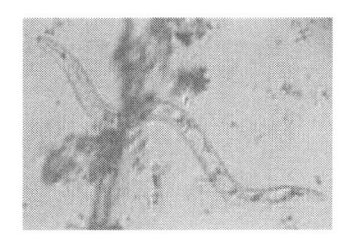

Roundworms are the most common intestinal parasite in the world, affecting over one billion people. They're also one of the largest parasites and can grow to up to thirty inches in length. Humans can contract a roundworm infection by eating improperly cooked meat or by handling dogs or cats infested with roundworms. Symptoms include loss of appetite, allergic reactions, coughing, abdominal pain, edema, sleep disorders, and weight loss.

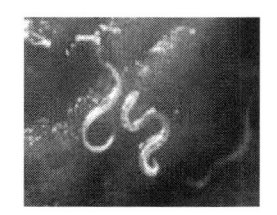

Hookworms are able to penetrate the human skin, and often enter the body through the feet when people walk barefoot through contaminated areas. They can be all over the world, especially in warm, moist tropical areas, and can live in the intestines for up to fifteen years. A hookworm infection may cause symptoms such as itchy skin, blisters, nausea, dizziness, anorexia, and weight loss.

Trichinella parasites, caused by the consumption of raw or undercooked pork, can mimic the symptoms of up to fifty different diseases. Possible symptoms of infection include muscle soreness, fever, diarrhea, nausea, vomiting, edema of the lips and face, difficulty breathing, difficulty speaking, enlarged lymph glands, and extreme dehydration.

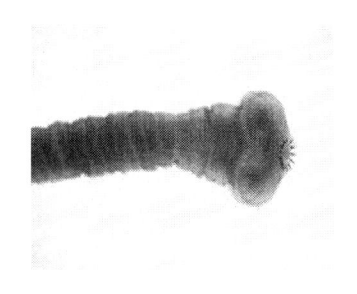

Tapeworms are the largest colon parasites that are known to infect humans. There are different types of tapeworms that infect different animals—there are beef tapeworms, pork tapeworms, fish tapeworms, and dog tapeworms. They can grow to several feet in length and live in the intestines for up to twenty-five years. Symptoms of a tapeworm infection are diarrhea, abdominal cramping, nausea, and change of appetite.

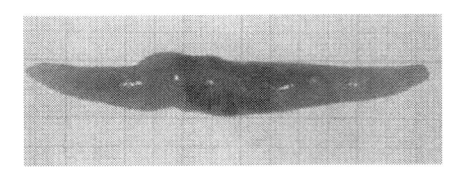

Flukes, or trematodas, are small flatworms that can penetrate the human skin when an individual is swimming or bathing in contaminated water. Flukes can travel throughout the body and settle in the liver, lungs, or intestines. Symptoms of a fluke infection include diarrhea, nausea, vomiting, abdominal pain, and swelling.

Avoiding Colon Parasites

You can reduce your risk of parasitic infection through simple, commonsense behaviors. Becoming vegetarian is a good start! By not eating meat, you avoid the common parasites that are passed on through undercooked food, and you won't have all of that slow-to-digest meat hanging around your colon and providing a breeding ground for toxic bacteria.

Wash your hands frequently. Carefully washing you hands several times throughout the day can remove the parasites and their eggs with which you may have come in contact. It's extra important to wash your hands after using the toilet, handling pets, cooking, or changing a baby's diaper, and before eating or handling food.

Avoid contaminated water. Unclean water is a common source of parasitic infection. Use bottled water for drinking or cooking if you don't trust the source of your water supply—and don't bathe in water that may be infested with parasites.

Wear shoes outdoors. Going barefoot is a pleasurable experience, but some colon parasites can enter the body through the soles of the feet. Be sure to wear shoes, especially if you are in an area like the beach or a park where there may be animal feces on the ground.

Wash and peel all fruits and vegetables. A quick scrub will remove parasites from fresh produce, and it's important that you do so before you eat them.

Brain-eating Worms

Some parasites can move to the human brain, and the results are quite horrible. It's not especially easy for a parasite to make it to the brain; a brain parasite's life does have its hardships. To begin with, the parasite has to find a way into the brain. There's a protective barrier between the bloodstream and the brain fluid, called the blood-brain barrier, that creates a tight seal so that substances from the bloodstream, including bacteria and parasites, don't leak into the brain. Even if a parasite does make it into the brain, it still has to battle the body's immune system, which attacks foreign bodies to protect us from harm. But some very tenacious parasites have found ways to fight back, evolving as tough warriors that can overcome the immune system. And these are the parasites that also do the most damage once they beat the odds.

Millions of people around the world are infected by brain parasites, mostly in nonindustrialized countries where sanitation is poor. Many of these brain parasites cause debilitating conditions, and sometimes death. One of the most debilitating of these is the pork tapeworm, *Taenia solium,* which is also one of the most common disease-causing brain parasites. Infecting over fifty million people worldwide, *Taenia solium* is the leading cause of brain seizures.

Usually contracted from eating undercooked pork, the parasite attaches itself to the intestine and grows several feet long. The especially tenacious worms that make it to the brain don't grow nearly that large, but they can do irreparable damage, even causing death. The risk to the brain comes when the eggs of these worms are swallowed. If ingested during their larval stage, the worms attach themselves to the intestine, but if eggs are swallowed, they hatch in the stomach and—for reasons that are still a mystery to researchers—can break through the blood-brain barrier and enter the brain. Some scientists believe that the larvae release enzymes that are able to dissolve enough of the blood-brain barrier to create a passage into the brain.

Once they reach the brain, the worms attach themselves to either the brain tissue or to cavities through which brain fluid flows; this causes a disease called neurocysticercosis resulting from formation of cysts in the brain by the parasites. The symptoms exhibited by victims of neurocysticercosis depend on the part of the brain in which the cysts form.

When attached to brain tissue, victims usually experience seizures. If the larvae attaches to the brain cavities, victims experience headaches, nausea, dizziness, and altered mental states (in addition to seizures!) because the flow of the brain fluid is blocked by the larvae. The lining of the brain cavities also become inflamed, further constricting the flow of the brain fluid and creating pressure on the brain. This increased pressure forces the heart to pump more blood to the brain, which increases the pressure even more. If left untreated, parts of the brain begin to die from a deficiency of blood, and serious brain damage occurs.

It can be a very slow process, often undetected for years. Many people play host to brain parasites for a long time before showing any symptoms. The worms have a sophisticated method of breaking down any antibodies in their vicinity and actually using them as a food source, effectively turning the body's tools for fighting them into a way for them to actually flourish!

One way to avoid contracting *Taenia solium* is to make sure that any pork you eat is thoroughly cooked. But an even better way to avoid these nasty, brain-eating worms is to become a vegetarian. Why play Russian roulette with the health of your brain when you can simply skip eating animal proteins entirely and get all your nutrition form a plant-based diet?

Cleaning Out the Pipes

One way to maintain colon health is to occasionally treat yourself to a colon cleansing. This can be administered by a professional, you can purchase herbal products designed for the purpose at a natural foods store, or you can ask a nutritionist to advise you on a good colon-cleansing method.

A colon cleanse isn't the same thing as an enema or dosing yourself with laxatives. There are drawbacks to both of those practices. Enemas, while fine when administered correctly on an occasional basis, can actually create as many problems as they solve. For example, if you use tap water, you may be injecting more parasites into your intestine. Enemas also only cleanse the larger, lower part of the intestine and do nothing to clean out the small intestine where many parasites dwell.

Laxatives may seem to be doing a great job of blowing out the pipes, but they're not effective in cleaning the small intestine and instead irritate the sensitive lining of the bowels. Overuse of laxatives leads to inefficient absorption of important nutrients; they act as a diuretic, increasing the risk of dehydration. The body can also become dependent on laxatives, ultimately causing more constipation than before.

Talk to your nutritionist or ask at your natural foods store for recommendations on doing a herbal colon cleanse. After flushing the toxin-producing parasites from your body, you'll feel much better!

CHAPTER 7

The Happy Vegetarian

How a Meatless Diet Will Improve Your Health and Well-Being

Overall health and well-being is a foreign concept to many people. They don't realize that they have the power to control their own health and that their well-being is often dependent on what they choose to eat and how active they allow themselves to be. Sooner or later, their bad choices catch up with them, and they end up overweight (or obese) with a multitude of health problems. They develop heart disease, diabetes, high cholesterol, and a slew of other deadly conditions that could have easily been avoided. All you have to do is be aware of what you are eating. There is more power on your dinner plate than you realize.

It is a known fact that vegetarians, as a whole, are more healthy that nonvegetarians. They have lower rates of cancer, high blood pressure, heart disease, gall bladder problems, and more. They also tend to be more active, involved, and aware of the environment because the principles of a vegetarian diet often permeate into other aspects of life. Lowered cholesterol, high amounts of vitamins, nutrients, and fiber, and a healthier lifestyle are all guaranteed benefits you will get simply by becoming a vegetarian.

Now, let's talk digestion, a topic that is both fascinating and important. If you still have any lingering suspicions that humans are supposed to eat meat as a primary source of protein, you might want to take a look at the digestive tract of true carnivores.

Meat is hard to digest, and it takes time for it to break down so that the nutrients can be used by the body. We've already talked about the differences between the teeth of carnivores (sharp and pointy for tearing flesh) and the teeth of plant-eaters (blunt and flat, like ours), and that's where digestion begins—in the mouth.

While you're chewing your food, the enzymes in your saliva begin the digestive process—the first step in breaking it down to its most usable form. After you swallow, the food moves on to your stomach, where it's dunked in a bath of hydrochloric acid that breaks it down further into a substance called chyme. Chyme travels from there to the digestive tract where it's slowly pushed through by contractions of the intestines called peristalysis. As it goes, tiny little hairlike fingers called villa absorb most of the nutrients from the chyme.

Finally, the almost completely digested food makes it to the colon, where water and some more vitamins and nutrients are absorbed from it before its exit through the rectum.

Meat—the Protein that Overstays Its Welcome

Here's where it gets interesting. Looking at a true carnivore—like, say, the lion with his big sharp teeth—we can see enormous differences in their digestive tract. Specifically, the lion's small intestine, are only about three times the length of his body. This means that the meat he eats moves through his system quickly, while it's still fresh.

Humans, however, have much longer intestines, with food taking anything from twelve to nineteen hours to pass through the digestive system. This is ideal for plant-based foods, as it allows our intestinal tracts to absorb every little bit of nutrient available, but it also means that when we eat meat it's decaying in a warm, moist environment for a very long time. As it slowly rots in our guts, the decaying meat releases free radicals into the body.

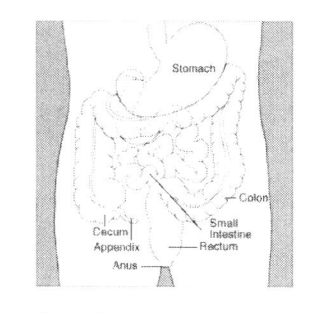

Free radicals are unstable oxygen molecules that are present to some degree in every body. When you hear advertisements trumpeting the importance of foods and supplements containing cancer-fighting antioxidants, it's these free radicals they're battling.

Scientists only know a little bit about free radicals at this time, but what they do know is that free radicals are connected with the aging process and that they may play a part in heart disease and cancer. They are, essentially, the tiny mechanisms that break down our bodies so that, eventually, we die.

While they'll always be a part of you—free radicals are built into cells as part of their normal activities—you can do things to minimize their damage. Overexposure to sunlight resulting in excessive tanning encourages the production of free radicals, which is why even though a little sunlight is important each day (remember our buddy, vitamin D?), using a good sun block will not only help you avoid skin cancers, it'll help keep you younger in general. But the biggest thing you can do to limit the free radicals in your body is to avoid eating meat. For the twelve hours or more that meat is rotting away in your system, those tiny, free radical time bombs are multiplying in your system.

As meat protein breaks down, it creates an enormous amount of nitrogen-based by-products, like urea and ammonia, which can cause a buildup of uric acid. Too much uric acid in your body leads to stiff, sore joints; when the uric acid crystallizes, it can cause gout and increased pain from arthritis. Carnivorous animals, interestingly, produce a substance called uricase, which breaks down uric acid. Humans don't produce uricase, though—another clue that we're not meant to be meat eaters.

The Raw and the Cooked

When you eat meat, how much of it do you eat raw? Well, Mr. Lion eats his raw, while it's still brimming with enzymes that aid in digestion. Humans, however, cook their meat. In fact, we cook our meat to temperatures over 130 degrees Fahrenheit. This has the benefit of killing most disease-causing bacteria, but it also kills the enzymes in the meat.

Whenever you eat dead food—-food lacking in the natural enzymes that help you digest it—your pancreas has to work extra hard to provide more so the food will break down for digestion. This puts strain on the pancreas that it wasn't originally designed to handle. This isn't to say that you should eat raw meat, like the lion. But it's another consideration when we look at whether humans are designed to eat meat; when true carnivores eat raw, fresh meat, all the enzymes are present to help them garner the nutrients they need as it passes quickly through their short digestive tracts, and the nutrient-depleted waste is eliminated soon after.

When we eat cooked meat, though, our bodies have to work extra hard to digest it by using precious energy needed for other purposes, overtaxing the pancreas, and creating free radicals as the dead flesh decays in our intestinal tract. But when we eat a plant-based diet, we're feeding ourselves food that's abundant with living enzymes, which break down efficiently in our systems and provide extra energy.

The Diabetic Vegetarian

The first line of combat when dealing with diabetes has always been diet. But with nutritionists and doctors radically changing their opinions on diabetics' best dietary options, research has been a hit-and-miss affair over the years. For a long time, it was believed that carbohydrates were the primary cause of diabetics; doctors would advise diabetic patients to limit their carbohydrate intake to just 20 percent of their total calories. Yet many cultures that maintain diets high in carbohydrates have much lower rates of diabetes than Western societies. So what's the deal?

Current research indicates that it's not carbohydrates that are the problem, it is the type of carbohydrates we eat. Simple carbohydrates, like those present in sugar and processed flour, raise the blood sugar so quickly that the pancreas has to create the hormone insulin to process it; complex carbohydrates, the kind found in fruits, vegetables, and whole grains, take longer to break down into glucose, so the body doesn't have the extreme insulin-producing reaction as with the simple sugars.

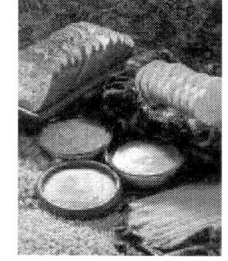

The American Diabetes Association now recommends that diabetics eat a diet that features a generous amount of slow-burning complex carbohydrates—including lots of fiber—with a moderate amount of protein and a low percentage of fat. Well, guess what? The vegetarian diet fits that prescription better than any other! In a study at the Pritikin Longevity Institute, a diet with 10 percent fat and just three ounces of meat per week was shown to radically help patients with type 2 diabetes, allowing many of the diabetics to stop using medication to treat the condition.

Slimming Down on a Vegetarian Diet

Believe it or not, there are fat vegetarians—just as there are thin people who eat a lot of red meat. It's possible to have a terrible diet that just happens to preclude animal proteins, and then there are complex issues of body type and metabolism as well. But there's still some truth to the stereotype. A vegetarian eating a healthy diet consisting of a wide array of whole foods is unlikely to be overweight, and so are those who eat meat now and then but subsist mainly on plant foods.

If your omnivorous lifestyle has left you with more pounds than you're comfortable with, then your new vegetarian diet is a great way to lose the extra weight. We've already talked about how the foods you eat provide your body with the various nutrients it needs to build strong bones, organs, skin, etc. And plant foods are easier to digest than animal foods. So, by taking up a vegetarian diet, you're saving energy that you can use to be more active. Most people who switch to vegetarian diets notice that there's more pep in their step because of the more efficient manner in which they're fueling their body. So use that extra energy to get up and get moving; it's an important step in weight control!

You'll also find that your appetite is under control on a vegetarian diet. When you feed your body foods rich in the nutrients it needs, in an easily digestible form, you won't find yourself with those mysterious cravings for more and more food at inappropriate times. When we eat a lot of animal foods, our colons become congested with mucus, toxins, and the detritus of decaying flesh; this limits the absorption of nutrients from our food.

Removing that blockage from the lower intestine is why many people swear by regular cleansing of their colon, either through professionally administered therapeutic enemas or by treating yourself to a do-it-yourself colon cleanser. Two or three weeks after transitioning to your vegetarian diet, mix a morning drink of apple juice with a tablespoon of aloe vera and liquid chlorophyll. Along with it, take two to four psyllium capsules and two capsules of cascara sagrada; these are readily available where nutritional supplements are sold. Be warned, though—this will have an invigorating effect on your bowels, so do it on a day that you're at home and close to the bathroom!

It's Not the Quantity, it's the Quality

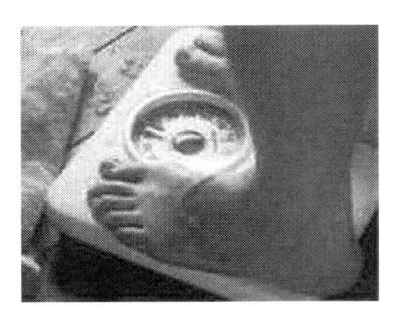

Weight loss diets for omnivores usually involve restricting something—fat, carbohydrates, or calories. These diets are great for losing weight quickly. But most people gain weight back after their initial weight loss for two reasons: their diet isn't something they can stay on for the rest of their lives, and extreme diets ultimately slow the metabolism.

Let's face it. Anyone can lose weight by cutting back on the amount of food they eat. It's called starvation! If you've ever been on a severely restrictive diet and felt cranky, light-headed, and low on energy, it's because your body wasn't getting the nutrients it needed. Burning stored fat is, of course, necessary for weight loss, but there are a lot of other things that you need from the food you eat just to get through the day. And eventually, restrictive diets actually have the result of making you fat.

Our bodies were ingeniously designed to survive in times of famine. When the eating's good, we store extra energy in the form of fat for later use. When the pickings are slim, however, and we're eating less than we need to survive, our bodies kick on the emergency backup system and burn the stored fat for energy. This worked brilliantly when man foraged for his food and ate whatever he could find—when he went for long periods with nothing to eat, he got thinner but he didn't die because of the stored fat reserves.

Your body does the same thing, even though you aren't foraging for food and going through long periods of famine. Every time you go on a restrictive diet, your body thinks that it's starving. So your metabolism slows down, burning less energy and keeping you alive in the face of starvation.

When you try to go back to eating normally your body leaps at the chance to store fat for the next time starvation comes, so you gain weight even faster than before. Your metabolism is slower, so you have less energy, you're less inclined to exercise, and your body holds onto what you give it for even longer.

So what's the solution? Eat healthy foods, in moderation, to keep your metabolism chugging along like a well-oiled machine. And stay away from the junk food—just because those chocolate-covered granola bars and cheese puffs are meat-free, that doesn't mean they're good dietary choices.

Now that you've successfully given up eating animal protein, take this opportunity to pick up other good habits too. Drink water instead sodas loaded with sugar (or aspartame). Satisfy your sweet tooth with fresh fruit instead of candy, eat whole-grain baked foods instead of white bread, and start using rice milk instead of dairy. Your body will thank you!

Feeling Good, Looking Good

There's truth to the adage, "you are what you eat." Once you start fueling your body with healthful foods, it'll show on the outside!

Take, for example, your skin. It's the body's largest organ and takes up about 12 percent of your body weight; it's also the first thing you present to the world. Your skin is alive—it breathes and needs moisture and the right nutrients to keep it not just blemish-free, but glowing and attractive. And it's arguably your most important organ of all; it keeps your muscles, organs, and bones protected from the elements.

The old, dry top layer of your skin sloughs off and is replaced every day or two. When you damage your skin, your body's system of self-repair is remarkable—you get a cut or scrape, and blood flows into the wound to flush out any foreign particles. Then your white blood cells go to work to fight infection, and nutrients like zinc and calcium kick in to build new skin cells to repair the damage. It's pretty amazing when you think about it.

You can repay all the good things your skin does for you by feeding it foods rich in the nutrients it craves. All plant foods contain a substance called bioflavinoids, which give plants' cells the solid structure they need. In the human body, bioflavinoids serve the same general purpose of nourishing the cells of your blood vessels. When these blood vessels, called capillaries, weaken and break, they leak blood and cause spider veins. These reddish splotches can appear anywhere on your body, particularly your cheeks, nose, and legs. By eating foods rich in bioflavinoids, you'll help to keep your blood vessels strong. Besides spider veins, weak blood vessels also lead to a variety of circulatory problems, including the tendency to bruise easily.

When it comes to looking your best, healthy skin is of vital importance. As an organ, one of skin's most important functions is to eliminate waste products through your perspiration. As with urine, the moisture that passes out of your body when you sweat carries with it the end product of the nutrients you didn't need for your bodily functions. Animal products contain very concentrated protein; when excess protein is filtered through the body, whatever your kidneys can't handle makes its way out of your body through your sweat. Some of it clogs your pores, making your skin dry and flaky and creating blemishes.

By eating a vegetarian diet, you won't be making your kidneys work so hard, you'll have less impurities passing through your skin, and you'll help the blood flow freely through your blood vessels. That glow of good health is the mark of a vegetarian!

The Sweet Scent of Good Health

We've talked about how eating meat clogs up the bowels and fills the body with toxins that it has trouble eliminating. Constipation is one side effect of this and happens when waste matter gets trapped in the intestinal tract. When that happens, toxins circulate throughout your body, looking for a way to get out; many of them end up in the lungs to be eliminated through your breath. This condition is called halitosis, in which no amount of mints can help reduce the foul smell in your breath.

Believe it or not, chronic bad breath can be eliminated by paying attention to the other end of things. Colon cleansing, which you'll remember from the chapter on nutrition, often clears up halitosis. Not that halitosis should be a problem if you're a vegetarian—all those healthy whole grains, fruits, and vegetables are loaded with fiber, and clogged bowels are an unlikely thing to happen.

But if you are yet to completely give up meat, you'll find your breath will be sweeter after its by-products are out of your body. And your whole body will smell better overall. When we eat meat, we're also eating whatever those animals ate, along with the various toxins stored in their fat. When you work out and burn your own stored fat, these toxins are sweated out through your skin. The less toxins you have in your body, the less your sweat and breath will smell.

Water In, Water Out

Almost every aspect of our body's functionality is regulated by hormones. When we eat meat, we ingest prostaglandins, hormonelike substances present in animal products as well as our own bodies. Excess prostaglandins can lead to an imbalance of your own hormone levels, which in its turn causes water retention.

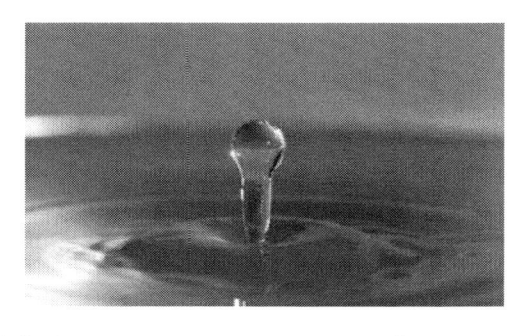

While nobody wants to be puffy—and when switching to a vegetarian diet, most people quickly see an improvement in their appearance because of decreased water retention—this is especially unpleasant when a woman is having, or is about to have, her menstrual cycle. Premenstrual syndrome, or PMS, is marked by inflammation, swelling, and bloating due to an excess of prostaglandins. If you're a woman and you've begun a vegan lifestyle, you're almost entirely assured that you'll see your symptoms of PMS diminish. If you're an ovo-lacto-vegetarian, try cutting out cheese and dairy during the week before you begin your period; this will give your hormones a breather so you can have a less uncomfortable cycle.

You'll find, as you get further into your vegetarian journey, that you look better, feel better, and even smell better. You'll also have more energy, which will help you be more active, and the more exercise you get, the better you'll look and feel. It's hard to believe that we're attractive when we feel lousy; our sluggish, fatigued bodies just drag along from meat-based meal to meat-based meal. But as a vegetarian, you'll have a spring in your step and a better outlook. How can you not feel good about yourself when you're eating healthy, socially responsible meals and treating yourself in the best way possible? So along with your shinier hair, clearer skin, and boosted energy, you'll radiate with the confidence that comes from taking excellent care of yourself—and that confidence is irresistible!

CHAPTER 8

"But I'm Not a Freak!" or, "How Do I Cope in a Carnivorous World?"

Being new to vegetarianism, it's more than likely that you're the only person in your household going meatless. Whether you live with a partner, your parents, your children, or roommates, sticking to your guns when everyone else is gorging on meat loaves or cheeseburgers can be difficult. Even if they're supportive of your decision, you'll have to deal with them not understanding all the ins and outs of your new lifestyle. And if they're not supportive, you may find them ridiculing your food choices or even actively trying to sabotage you.

The first thing you need to accept is that it's not your job to make them change to suit your way of eating any more than it's theirs to turn you back into a meat eater. If they want to change, that's great. You can share this book with them, and you can all work on menu planning together! But the best way you can influence others in your household to adopt healthier habits is to be a good example—and not turn them off by lecturing them!

Mealtime at an Omnivorous Dinner Table

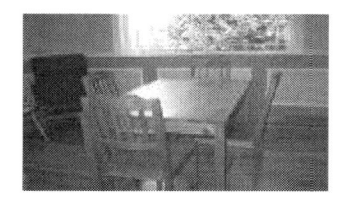

What's the best way to deal with vegetarian needs when the rest of the family expects meat and potatoes for dinner? Should you just partake of the same meal as the others, only skipping the meat? Or should you make it clear that you have special needs and eat a meal separate from everyone else's? If you're the primary cook in your family, you may not want to prepare multiple dishes every night, and you may not want to cook a meat-based dish for others when you've given it up yourself. And if you're not the family chef, is it fair to ask them to go to extra effort for you, night after night?

Only you know the dynamics in your home, so only you can figure out the answers to these questions. One thing is certain: you need to sit down and talk to the people you live with about your dietary needs and figure out the most agreeable way to make it work for everyone. If you can't stand to have meat around you at all, this is a huge issue. You may have to ask the others in your home to cook meat outside on a grill, dedicate a special section of the refrigerator to meat storage, and ask for it to be wrapped in such a way that you don't have to look at it. If your feelings aren't that strong, you may simply want to negotiate who cooks what, and when; perhaps you can arrange to cook completely vegetarian meals for everyone three nights a week and prepare your own entrée on the other nights. It all comes down to what your needs are and the compromises you and your family are willing to make.

What about the Children?

A little patience and negotiation can overcome issues between a nonvegetarian and a vegetarian, but what if you have children? It's a little like a mixed marriage where you have to decide in which religion you'll raise your children! Few areas can lead to disharmony in a relationship faster than disagreements on how to bring up the kids, so sit down and negotiate this one with your partner before you go any further.

Raising your child to be vegetarian is certainly a healthful option. Kids benefit from going meatless just like adults, and we'll discuss the how-to of that in chapter 17. The most important thing right now is to figure out how you'll handle meals at home with your kids. Some families eat nothing but meatless meals at home, but they allow the children to eat meat at school and at their friends' houses. Others create meals that offer options for everyone in the family, so that the omnivores and the vegetarians can choose whatever they like.

On the other hand, you may feel so strongly that your children become vegetarians that there may be no room for compromise. You'll need to lay this out for your partner in a kind, nonconfrontational way, but, even if you do, it may lead to conflict. It may seem like it is just food, but it's an important issue. If you can't easily negotiate the issue, there's no shame in working it out with a family counselor. Remember, though, that no matter what their age, people like to eat good food, so if you put together tasty, attractive menus full of flavor, color, and a variety of textures, you'll find that the kids and adults are more willing to try vegetarian meals.

Involving the Whole Family

Incorporating your vegetarian diet into your entire family's diet can be a bit of a challenge, especially if they do not want to change their eating habits. Trying to force your vegetarian eating style onto them will never work. Your spouse and your children will end up resenting the pressure and will refuse to try anything new. Instead of pushing your family, try some reverse psychology. Make irresistible and tasty vegetarian dishes that they can have the option to try. If the dish tastes good to them, they will want more of it. For example, put a bowl of pasta topped with vegetarian marinara sauce on the dinner table next to a bowl of pasta with meat sauce. See which bowl empties the fastest. After a few more dinners like this, you will eventually be making nothing but vegetarian meals. And the rest of your family may not even notice the difference.

Another way of incorporating vegetarian dishes into your family meal plan is by starting with simple vegetarian choices that most people enjoy. For example, everyone loves stir-fry. Make it with assorted vegetables and serve it over steamed rice. Cook the chicken or beef separately, and leave it up to the rest of your family to decide whether or not they would like to add meat to their dish.

Other vegetarian dishes that can be served to meat eaters include:

    Bean burritos
    Vegetarian chili
    Pasta primavera
    Italian stuffed shells

Vegetable jambalaya
Vegetable soup
Pesto pasta

The important thing to remember is that every family is different. Talk to the members of your family, and learn what kinds of food they enjoy. Be willing to compromise in order to keep everyone complacent. After all, you wouldn't want someone telling you what you should or shouldn't be eating. Keep this in mind when seeking your family's support. Once you find out what vegetarian meals they are willing to eat, make those on a regular basis before introducing new ones into the mix. You can also get the entire family involved by including them in on the meal planning. Have them choose vegetarian recipes that they will enjoy, and let them have some input on how to keep both the vegetarians and nonvegetarians in the family happy. Grow some vegetables together, shop together, and cook together. Making vegetarian meals can be a fun learning experience for everyone.

It all basically comes down to this: don't push! Instead, teach by example. If your family isn't ready to make the switch from carnivore to herbivore, then do it yourself without making a fuss. Chances are, with time, the rest of the members of your family will notice what you are doing and may eventually follow in your footsteps. We all have our own family have the opportunity and ability to make food choices to make. So let your choices be their choices as well. The right approach and attitude can make all the difference in the world.

If you're the main cook in the family, preparing multiple entrees for family dinners can be a lot of extra work, but it's also the easiest solution to making sure you get something to eat while keeping everyone happy. And, you'll be surprised to learn, it's also the best way to sway others to your side.

Look at it this way: your omnivorous tablemates can enjoy the meat-based portion of the meal while you eat your vegetarian option, and all of you can share the vegetarian side dishes. Of course, your vegetarian food is going to look so good and smell so delicious, they'll want to try your food too. So the next time, you just make the vegetarian dish, and chances are they'll never miss the meat-based dish! Pretty soon, you'll be making vegetarian meals almost every day of the week ... mission accomplished.

You can also make your meal out of all of the nonmeat dishes on the table, which (if you plan well) should be enough to fill up your plate and your belly. Steamed vegetables, roasted red potatoes, a salad, and a whole-wheat roll is a fine meal; let the others have the pork chops, because you've got plenty to eat. This is a good approach when you find yourself at a Thanksgiving dinner, office party, or dinner at a friend's house and you can't dictate the menu; just eat what you can, without making a big deal out of your vegetarian lifestyle.

You and Me against the World

Right now, as you start your new vegetarian life, you can decide what sort of a vegetarian you're going to be. And the best way to decide that is to think about all of the people you've known in your life who have tried to convert you to their personal way of living.

We all know the type. The two-pack-a-day smoker who gives up cigarettes and then lectures everyone within earshot on the dangers of second-hand smoke. The born-again Christian who drops the Lord's name into every conversation and acts as a self-proclaimed expert on morality. The former boozehound that takes the 12 Steps so seriously that you can't even swallow an antihistamine in their presence without getting an earful about addiction.

And you know what? We really, really don't like those people. So don't become one!

You've made an important life choice that's going to improve most areas of your life, most notably your health. And it will be tempting to loudly proclaim to everyone around you about how great vegetarianism is—after all, you've made positive changes that would benefit everyone, right? The problem is, most people are turned off by in-your-face proselytizing, and you'll do more to drive them away from the idea of meatless eating than you will to convert them. That's not to say that you shouldn't be honest about your choices, but badgering your friends and family takes it a step too far.

Some of the most influential people in the world have been those who quietly lived their lives by their own principles and inspired others to choose similar paths by example. Others will ask questions about your vegetarianism, and you should definitely be prepared to answer those questions. But if you find yourself continually battling with other people, arguing with them about your choices, and creating bad feelings, then you need to take a good, hard look at how you're getting across your message.

The Big Why

Your co-workers, family, friends, and even people you meet socially will have questions about your vegetarianism. The questions are wide-ranging, but they're all probably the same questions that you had when you first started this journey:

"How do you get enough protein if you don't eat meat?"
"What do you eat?"
"Do you eat chicken (or fish, or eggs)?"
"Don't you miss meat?"
"Can you still have dessert?"
"Why do you wear leather shoes?"
"Why can't you drink milk?"

…and so on. The best way to deal with these questions is to have a simple, honest answer ready. You're not required to go into detail about every aspect of your diet, and it's best if you don't—unless someone is really curious about those details. Don't try to sell them on vegetarianism. Just answer the questions, smile, and move on.

There's an old show business axiom that goes, "Always leave 'em wanting more." When people ask you about your vegetarianism, they're curious about what's so great about it. The happier, more secure, and more nonjudgmental about other people's eating that you are, the more they'll suspect that there's something valuable in it. Your answers will make them want to find out more, so they'll seek out more information. You may even be the one they come to, looking for advice.

In essence, you're an ambassador for vegetarianism. You know how better your new lifestyle is for you, the planet, and the animals. But that doesn't mean you have to act superior. If you have a positive, happy, low-key attitude toward your food choices, that will affect the way that people see not just you, but vegetarianism, too.

Support is Key

Surrounding yourself with likeminded vegetarians is key. There is always power in numbers. And when you surround yourself with positive reinforcement, you will be less likely to revert back to your nonvegetarian ways.

If you happen to live in a large city, there are probably numerous local vegetarian support groups lurking around every corner. Use the Internet to locate one of these groups and attend a meeting. You may feel like an outsider at first, but once you talk and listen to other members of the group who were once in your shoes, you will feel more at home. Most meetings are informal and revolve around discussions of transition, tips, recipes, personal struggles, and the positive impact that vegetarianism has on the world as a whole. Try using meetup.com, a great forum for local groups to recruit members and connect through the Internet. There are a variety of vegetarian-themed groups that will help you meet like-minded individuals in your area. (You can also join veggie123.com discussion forums.)

You can become an active member of one of the many national vegetarian organizations across the country. Though they function quite differently than local organizations, they can still offer some form of support. Sign up for their monthly newsletter (if they have one) or visit their Web site and join the forum. Interacting with other vegetarians is the best way to get acclimated to your new way of thinking and eating. Attend a national conference and listen to speakers from all over the country who can offer expert advice and address issues regarding vegetarianism.

I would advise you to join both a local and national organization as you continue on with your transition. Even after you are comfortable with your vegetarian lifestyle, it helps to stay connected to a vegetarian network to maintain a sense of synergy and well-being. The local organization can keep you up-to-date about what's going on in your neck of the woods, while the national organization will give you a larger perspective.

If you can't find a local support group near you, pay a visit to an alternative health care center. These particular centers often pride themselves on holistic healing traditions, which sometimes include vegetarianism. Most alternative health care centers are associated with hospitals or counseling centers. You local health food store can also point you in the right direction. Health fairs can also offer numerous resources as well.

Treading Gently on the Earth and on Other People's Feelings

You'll have countless experiences in the coming years where you're surrounded by people eating meat, and where maintaining a vegetarian lifestyle is a challenge. You may be on a road trip with friends, and the only place to eat is a fast-food burger joint. Or a family picnic turns out to be a nonstop barbecue with the main fare consisting of burgers, hot dogs, and ribs. In these situations, your only option is to find whatever you can to eat—a glass of apple juice or diet soda, a handful of potato chips, or some coleslaw—and make the best of the situation.

This won't happen very often, because vegetarians really do have a wide range of food choices, but when it does, it's up to you to behave with dignity. Eat what you can, and show how adaptable you are. This will not only show them what a charming, mature, and flexible person you are, it'll also give them a good impression of vegetarianism as a whole. Remember, most nonvegetarians fear that switching to a meatless lifestyle will be boring and difficult. By showing them that it's not, you're soft selling vegetarianism.

If you're dining out with a mixed group of vegetarians and nonvegetarians, do what you can to get everyone to agree on a restaurant that has plenty of vegetarian options. If these are family members or close friends (as opposed to, say, a business function), you can even ask politely if everyone would be okay with eating somewhere that has menu items for vegetarians—it's likely that they'll accommodate you with a minimum of grumbling.

If you're vegan, the challenge will be even greater, and you'll find that you have to be the most adaptable of all. While most restaurants today plan their menus with an eye toward offering vegetarian options, few offer much—if anything—for vegans. You'll find that you have to make do when dining out, especially with a mixed group that includes nonvegetarians. But the important thing is to do it with grace and not draw undue attention to your special dietary needs.

In fact, some vegetarians make special allowances for times that they have absolutely no control over the food that's available and will eat foods made with eggs or dairy. This way, they can socialize with nonvegans without going hungry or risking negative interactions because of their dietary restrictions. It's not the ideal way to live as a vegan, of course, but we live in an imperfect world. The most important thing is to stay true to your principles, as much as you realistically can, and inspire others to see vegetarianism as a positive, flexible lifestyle. Remember, the more attractive you make it look, the more likely it is that they'll want to try it themselves!

Allow Yourself Time to Get Healthy

Hopefully, you haven't been overwhelmed by all the information you've read thus far. It's a lot to digest (so to speak) about nutrition. It's important to have a basic grasp of what your body needs to function properly, but it's also important to remember that if you eat a variety of whole foods each day, then you're undoubtedly getting enough nutrients. Feeling confident that you're eating well as a vegetarian will be give you strength to deal with nonvegetarians who don't understand what your choice is all about—or, even worse, have a head full of misinformation that they're so convinced is the truth, they'll argue with you.

The first line of psychological defense in a world of carnivores is this one thought: vegetarian diets are not lacking in essential nutrients any more than nonvegetarian diets. Which isn't to say that all vegetarians eat well. Just like omnivores, some vegetarians have absolutely horrible diets. And the culprit in both cases is usually the same thing: junk food.

By switching to a vegetarian lifestyle, you've become much more thoughtful about what you eat. But that doesn't mean you're immune to the siren call of junk food like chocolate chip cookies, salty chips, and soft drinks. Even if you shop primarily at a natural foods store, you'll find the aisles are lined with convenience foods and snacks— including even cookies and chips marketed to vegans! It's natural to want a treat every now and then, or to fall back on prepackaged foods when we're short on time. The problem rises when you find that commercially prepared foods are equal in amount or are outnumbering the meals that you make from scratch.

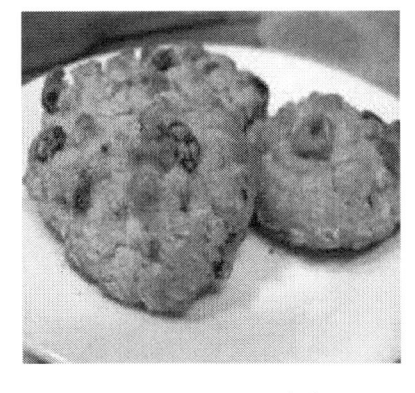

Our lives are all busy, and we have so much that we have to manage— family responsibilities, jobs, and social obligations. Usually we place our own needs at the bottom of our list of priorities. Often, we feel selfish about taking time out for ourselves when we have so much we need to do and so many places we need to be. Meals get short shrift because we just can't be bothered to chop and slice and simmer and bake. If you're not a naturally talented chef, you may not get pleasure out of cooking, and you just want to get it on the table so you can eat and get back to other things on your priority list.

Keep in mind that one of the reasons that you've chosen a new way of eating is to have more control over what you put into your body. Processed health foods from commercial vendors still contain salt, sugar, and fat, and when you rely on them, you're losing a lot of control over what you eat. You also may find yourself buying foods based entirely on how good they taste rather than how healthy they are.

Tracking Your Success

It's possible to lose track of what you're eating, especially if you're very busy. If you think that you may be relying too much on processed foods, carry a small notebook with you and make it your food diary for a week. Write down everything you eat, when you eat it, and how much. At the end of the week, you'll have a good idea of where your danger areas are, which less healthy foods you're eating too much of, and even what times of the day you reach for snacks. It's good information to have, and it can help you change some potentially self-sabotaging habits.

Meanwhile, help yourself out by planning ahead. We'll talk about stocking your kitchen and planning meals in chapter 12, but for now, think about ways that you can streamline the system for cooking at home. Prepackaged salads, fruits, and vegetables are more expensive than those you buy in the produce section and prepare yourself, but if you find yourself skipping these important foods—in the lunch that you bring to work, for example—because of the time it takes to prepare them, consider trading the extra money they cost for the time you'll save. Another solution is to take a little time when you grocery shop to wash and cut up a variety of fruits and vegetables as soon as you bring them home, and store them in airtight plastic containers and Ziploc bags so they're ready to go when you need them. Some companies make small snack-size bags that are perfect for cut-up carrots, celery, and fruit, so you can just grab a bag of snacks to take with you whenever you leave the house (and if you're concerned about adding plastic to the landfill, you can always rinse them out and reuse them later).

Of course, you're going to want cookies or cake or chips every once in a while. You're only human! It's also possible to eat healthy by incorporating frozen vegetarian meals, vegan snack bars, and vegetarian cup of soup-type items into your diet. But if you look at your cupboards and see a preponderance of sweet treats, salty snacks, and instant meals, it's time to take a step back and reassess how much of your diet is made up of whole foods and how much is junk.

Hide and Seek—Identifying Hidden Animal Products

So you've stopped eating meat, and you're feeling good about being a vegetarian. You know that you've chosen an ethical, thoughtful, healthy way of life, and you've mastered the art of meatless eating. But are you really eliminating all animal products from your diet?

Many, many commercially produced foods contain ingredients from animal sources. Some of these ingredients can be produced from plant sources, but unless a manufacturer specifies the source on the label, you have no way of knowing if its origins are animal. Often, these are additives that are derived from eggs or dairy products and are thus acceptable to ovo-lacto-vegetarians. But if you're vegan, you have to be especially careful about reading labels; animal products can be found in the most unlikely of places.

Albumin is the protein in eggs—specifically, egg whites. It's often used as a thickening agent.

Anchovies, those tiny, salty fish that you pick off your pizza, are an ingredient in Caesar salad dressing and Worcestershire sauce.

Animal fats like butter, lard, and suet are used to make packaged crackers and cookies, as well as frozen piecrusts, refried beans, and flour tortillas.

Carmine, has a red coloring and is often found in juices, colored pasta, and candy. It's made from ground-up insects.

Casein, also listed as caseinate, is a milk protein added to cheese products and can even be found in some soy cheese.

Gelatin, used to thicken processed foods, is usually of animal origin; it is obtained from boiling down bones and cartilage. It's found in gelatin desserts, yogurt, candies, and sugar-coated cereals.

Glucose and dextrose, both simple sugars, can be derived from fruit but often comes from animal tissues and fluids. It's an ingredient in many soft drinks, baked foods, candies, and commercial frostings.

Glycerides are listed as monoglycerides, diglycerides, or triglycerides, and can be derived from either animal fats or from plant sources. They're found in a staggering number of products, from processed foods and cosmetics to hand lotions, ink, glue, and antifreeze.

Isinglass, a gelatin made from the air bladders of freshwater fish, is used as a clarifying agent in some gelatin-based desserts and alcoholic beverages.

Lactic acid is a milk-based bacteria used in cheese, yogurt, candies, jams and jellies, frozen treats, and processed vegetables like pickles, olives, and sauerkraut.

Lactose, sometimes listed as D-lactose or saccharin lactin, is the sugar found in milk. It's used as a sweetener in candies, over-the-counter medications, laxatives, baby formula, and as a culture medium in yogurts and sour cream.

Lactylic Stearate is salt of stearic acid and is used as a product in bread dough.

Lanolin is the fat in sheep's wool, and it's present in a wide range of cosmetics and lotions, as well as chewing gum and fabric treatments.

Lard should be avoided at all costs. It is made from the abdomen of pigs and is often used in baked foods and desserts as well as refried beans.

Lecithin, a necessary nutrient, is derived from both plant and animal sources, but it is most often derived from egg yolks. You'll see it in many products, including processed breakfast foods, margarine, baked foods, vegetable oil sprays, and chocolate.

Lutein, a yellow coloring agent, is made from either plant sources (marigolds) or animal sources (egg yolks) and is used to color a wide range of foods.

Oleinic acid, derived from sheep and cattle fat, is used in butter substitutes, cheese, vegetable oils, baked foods, candies, ice cream and beverages, as well as cosmetics and soap.

Pepsin, an enzyme from pigs' stomachs, is used to make cheese.

Stearic acid, also listed as octadecanoic acid, is derived from animal fat and is found in countless processed foods including baked foods, chewing gum, beverages, artificial vanilla flavoring, cosmetics, and the outer coating of pills.

Tallow, the waxy solid fat from sheep and cattle, is an ingredient in waxed paper, soap, margarine, crayons, and candles.

Vitamin A, also listed as retinol, can be derived from plant sources or from cod liver oil or egg yolks. It is used to fortify foods and is an old supplement on its own. It's also sometimes found in cosmetics.

Vitamin B12, another popular supplement, can be made from animal sources or synthesized. The synthetic version is vegan; look for "cobalymin" on the label.

Vitamin D comes in several forms and is used as a fortifying supplement. Vitamin D2, also listed as ergocalciferol, is derived from plant sources or yeast; vitamin D3, also identified as cholecalciferol, is made from cod liver oil or lanolin.

Whey, the liquid that's separated from milk solids when making cheese, can be found in many processed foods, especially baked foods.

Marching to Your Own Drummer

You'll soon find, as you identify yourself to others as a vegetarian, that there's a schoolyardlike rivalry among the vegetarians. Many vegans look down their noses at ovo-lacto-vegetarians, disapproving of their use of dairy and eggs and recoiling at the thought of their leather shoes. Avid ovo-lactos feel superior to semi-vegetarians who eat fish or chicken and think they aren't serious enough about vegetarianism.

It's all very petty, and being judgmental doesn't do anyone any good. Really, how you choose to eat is a very personal decision. You're taking the time to learn about nutrition and vegetarian styles and figuring out what works for you; don't let anyone bully you into feeling like you're not vegetarian enough. As you go along your vegetarian journey, you may find you want to become vegan, or semi-vegan, or whatever the next step is. Your diet will evolve as you go, depending on your needs.

Remember that only 1 percent of the entire population is vegetarian. You're going up against some very extreme odds and are functioning in a world that is based primarily on meat consumption. You are different from others but for very good reasons. You are choosing a path less traveled and that is something that should be celebrated. *You are deciding what kinds of foods you want to eat based on what is* healthiest for *your* body. Therefore, you don't owe anyone anything, and you certainly don't need to explain or justify your actions.

As a vegetarian, whatever stripe you are, you're going to be in the minority. Nitpicking over which subcategory is better is silly. Take pride in your specialness; after all, unlike most omnivores, you've put a lot of thought into this! You don't have to justify your choice to anyone. Be proud of yourself for deciding to feed yourself in a way that's healthier, more ethical, and more socially responsible. Being different doesn't mean you're a freak.

You're smart! You've proven yourself to be someone who thinks about how their choices affect their body and the rest of the world. Stand tall!

CHAPTER 9

The Vegetarian Eats Out
Meals You Can Enjoy, from Fast Food to Fine Dining

When you're making your own meals at home, it's easy to have complete control over every aspect of your eating. You stock the pantry, you plan the menus, and you whip up tasty vegetarian entrees for yourself and your family. But unless you're completely housebound, you have to go out in the world some time—and often, that requires eating in restaurants.

That doesn't mean you have to toss out all your vegetarian principles. Restaurants are increasingly offering vegetarian options, and even fast-food outlets have food you can eat. Depending on where you are, you can find something to eat. The reason restaurants have become more sensitive to the needs of vegetarians has nothing to do with social consciousness—it is all about money. Vegetarians (and friends of vegetarians) have money to spend, too, and restaurants that don't cater to vegetarian eaters lose business when those folks want to eat out.

Even if you end up in a restaurant that doesn't have anything vegetarian on the menu, you can always request something special. Remember, restaurants want your money, and they get that money by selling you food and preparing it in a way you like! Salads can be made without the chicken or salmon that's listed on the menu. You can even ask your server if the chef can prepare something vegetarian just for you. Chefs often get a little bored making the same things day in and day out, and yours may welcome the opportunity to whip up something new! Just be polite, ask nicely, and your request will be seen as perfectly reasonable.

Think Ethnic

If you live in a big city, you'll probably be able to find vegetarian restaurants in your town. If you can't find any on the Internet or in the phone book, look for a natural foods store in your town; the employees there will be able to point you toward restaurants that are vegetarian-friendly. If both of those searches come up short, think ethnic! Chinese restaurants are great for vegetarians, offering delicious vegetable entrees, rice, and noodles. Just take a moment to quiz your server about how the dishes are prepared—some dishes that sound vegetarian on the menu may contain meat or eggs. Tell your server that you don't eat meat, and they'll make sure your meal comes the way you want it.

Indian restaurants are terrific for vegetarians, too, although not all cities have them. The Indian diet has a rich tradition of vegetarianism, and restaurants offer a selection of vegetable curries and dishes made with chickpeas, which are an excellent source of protein (and delicious). If you're new to Indian cuisine, you have a delightful adventure ahead of you—try dal, a traditional, spicy lentil dish, and samosas, delightful little pastries stuffed with meat, vegetables, and spices (just make sure you don't order the ones with meat!). If you're avoiding dairy, be aware that many Indian dishes are prepared using clarified butter, called ghee; just ask that your meal be prepared with vegetable oil instead.

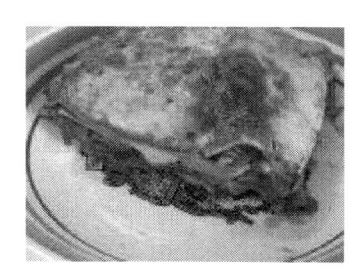

If your co-workers or family announce a trip to the Olive Garden or another Italian restaurant, don't fret. Italian restaurants are another great option for vegetarians, especially the ovo-lactos. Pasta with meatless marinara sauce is a staple menu item, as is pasta primavera, which is loaded with vegetables. Many Italian soups, such as pasta fagioli, contain protein from rice and beans (just make sure that they use vegetable broth and not beef or chicken). At the big chain restaurants like Olive Garden or the Spaghetti Factory, you'll find salad bar/bread stick combination meals that are perfect for vegetarians and easy on the wallet. And if the gang heads out for pizza, ovo-lactos have lots of options too. Plain cheese pizza, or even a cheeseless pizza topped with vegetables, is just as tasty as the meat-loaded kind.

Other ethnic options are excellent choices for vegetarians, as well. Hit a Greek restaurant and load up on hummus, dolma (stuffed grape leaves), baba ganoujh (a delicious eggplant spread), Spanikopita (spinach pie), and salad made with a grain called tabouli. If you like Mexican fare, you can have gazpacho (a cold vegetable soup), *chiles rellenos* (green peppers stuffed with cheese, then breaded and fried), and bean-and-cheese versions of all the usual favorites—burritos, enchiladas, tostadas, and tacos.

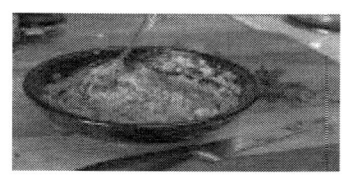

Eating with the Common Folk

If you're an ovo-lacto-vegetarian, you'll be able to find lots of things to eat at family-style restaurants, no matter what time of the day you visit them. At breakfast, you can enjoy waffles or pancakes, omelets, and egg scrambles. Other times of the day or night, there are grilled cheese sandwiches, salads, French fries, egg salad, and other items. It gets harder, however, if you're vegan. In fact, despite the size of the menus in these restaurants, vegans will find little that they can eat. This is where it pays to be creative and flexible. Ask your server if the kitchen will top a baked potato with steamed vegetables, or ask if you can just have a small salad, some veggies, and rice. It may not be the most delicious meal you've ever had, but it's an adequate meal until you can get something tastier.

As mentioned earlier in the chapter, your better restaurants will have menu items designed with vegetarians in mind, and even if there's nothing that's just what you want, the chef will probably be amenable to customizing a dish to your liking. Most of the time, though, you'll find delicious vegetarian appetizers—you can even make a meal out of two or three of those if there's no entrée that appeals to you. But you'd be surprised how creative a chef can be when asked to come up with something new on the spur of the moment, and your nonvegetarian friends will be jealous of the special attention you receive!

Vegetarians on the road

Traveling can be a special challenge when you're vegetarian, since you don't know what will be available to you ahead of time. It helps to be prepared for the worst and anticipate how you'll eat if there's little or nothing available for vegetarians; you'll need to be adaptable no matter what happens.

Car trips can be difficult if you rely on restaurants and fast food as your primary dining options. There are three very good reasons why you should make your own food to travel with: saving time, saving money, and eating healthy. By packing a cooler with your own food, you can control what you eat and when. Besides saving you the time you would spend looking for a vegetarian-friendly restaurant, you're assured that you can eat foods that fit with your vegetarian lifestyle. And you'll save money too—packing your own food is always less expensive than eating out.

Take a look at the foods you have on hand and consider how well they can be carried along on a road trip. Bring a cooler for the perishable items, and pack up a small box with the rest. Just be careful if you're eating while driving so you don't cause an accident! Here are some foods that are as tasty on the road as they are at home:

> Whole-grain muffins, rolls, and cookies
> Carrot sticks and celery
> Snack-size containers of yogurt, applesauce, and breakfast cereal
> Juice boxes
> Peanut butter (or almond butter) sandwiches
> Pasta salads
> Egg salad sandwiches
> Bagels
> Hummus and pita chips
> Trail mix

Fresh fruit
Vegan snack bars
Bottles of mineral water

When you're packing for a car trip, don't forget the little extras that will make your roadside meals hassle-free. Get a bag or box, and stock plastic utensils, paper plates, napkins, or paper towels, a bottle opener, a knife for slicing fruits and vegetables, Ziploc Baggies for leftovers, a gallon jug of water for rinsing off food and your hands, and some disposable wipes for easy cleanup. Consider keeping your toothbrush and toothpaste easily accessible so you can brush after your meal!

If you're into hiking or biking, make sure to pack foods that are easily portable and don't have to be refrigerated. You'll also want to pack foods that are rich in nutrients and provide you with lots of energy. Trail mix, dried fruits, vegetarian snack bars, Fig Newtons, crackers, and peanut butter are all good food choices. They will help keep you energized while you walk or bike to you destination.

Remember that the key to a healthy vegetarian diet is variety. Every meal doesn't have to be an entrée and side dishes—some granola, a single-serving container of rice milk, fresh fruit, and a whole-grain muffin makes a great meal! Munch on foods that you like during the day, and then spend your vacation money on a nice meal at dinnertime.

Flying High and Meat-free

Depending on what airline you fly and how long your trip is, your in-flight meal is likely to be a cellophane-wrapped package of crackers or a bag of pretzels. But some flights still serve meals and offer the option of a vegetarian snack. If you travel frequently and use a travel agent, you can let them know that you're vegetarian, and they'll make the request for you every time they book your flights. If you book your own flights, you simply need to make the request when you make your reservations or call the airline's customer service number (you can also visit their Web site) and make the request at least twenty-four hours before you're scheduled to fly.

If you're unsure if your flight will serve a meal, call and ask an airline representative; if you're vegan, make sure to specify no eggs or dairy.

Once you've made the request, call the day before your flight just to be certain that they have you down as vegetarian. When you board the plane, let the flight attendant know as soon as you can that you're getting a vegetarian meal—as with any bureaucracy, information is sometimes inefficiently communicated.

Occasionally, planes are changed at the last minute due to mechanical issues, and that can mean that your meal isn't loaded on the right plane! Then the same holds true if you upgrade to first class just before you board—they may have your meal ear-marked for your original seat assignment. Requesting a vegetarian meal is no guarantee that you'll get one, but by politely reminding the flight crew that you've made the request, you increase the odds that you'll get it.

Ahoy, Captain, There's a Vegetarian on Board!

When you are trapped on a big sailboat or cruise ship, food choices are limited. After all, you can ask the crew or the captain to pull over at the next port so that you can find some better vegetarian options. Luckily, cruises these days are all about luxury and accommodating the passengers. You are bound to find numerous vegetarian options on board for every meal. Some high-end cruises even offer a vegetarian menu for you to choose from. When you are dining on the cruise ship, you can always ask your server if a certain meat dish can be made without any meat products. Handle it just as you would if you were dining out. Ask for specifics on how the dish is made and inquire as to whether you can have your dish made vegetarian-style. The chef will most likely be more than happy to accommodate your needs.

When you are planning your cruise or boat outing, have your travel agent inquire about any specific dietary requests—such as a vegetarian meal plan. That way you will know what kind of situation you are getting into even before you step foot on the boat. Most cruise ships these days offer elaborate buffets that are piled high with calorie-rich foods and meats that vegetarians steer away from. But you are more than likely to find vegetarian options along the buffet line. Visit the salad area, fruit section, and bread table first to find vegetarian friendly foods. Then circle back around to see if there are any vegetables and pasta salads being served along side meat selections. While other passengers fret over the amount of weight they are gaining on the ship, you will find comfort in your vegetarian way of life once you put on your bathing suit to swim in the ocean!

Emergency Rations—The Vegetarian's Safety Net

Anyone who has special dietary needs, vegetarian or otherwise, should know how to put together a small pack of just-in-case food for those times when you'd otherwise be unable to get a healthy meal. This is a great idea for vegetarians, but it's vital for people with insulin problems—diabetics, prediabetics, and hypoglycemics—so they can keep their blood sugar in check.

Small, insulated lunch bags are ideal for this purpose. You want to be able to take it with you in your carry-on bag on air flights (check the current FAA rules regarding what you can, and can't, take on a plane) or toss in the car when you're going to be away from home all day.

Some things you can consider as emergency meal rations:

> Presliced vegetables like celery, carrots, bell peppers, and jicama
> Single-serve boxes of rice milk and/or fruit juice
> Sliced cheese
> Protein bars
> Apple slices
> Trail mix
> Snack packs of hummus and pita chips
> Bottled water
> Small container of peanut butter
> Chips or pretzels
> Bagels

If you're traveling, make sure you restock your emergency pack as you go along. Pick up granola bars, nuts, and chips from convenience stores and vending machines. If your hotel has a free continental breakfast, nab a piece of fruit for the bag.

Keeping your just-in-case bag stocked will save you time looking for something to eat and the money you'd spend for a restaurant or fast-food meal, and it'll be a life saver if you're stuck somewhere without anything available.

You Want Fries with That?

Fast food is difficult to avoid. Unless you live in a remote location miles from civilization or you never leave your house, you drive past fast-food outlets several times every day. And if you're out and about, or on the road in a strange town, they're an attractive option for a quick meal. But do they have anything that you can eat?

Thankfully, the answer is yes. Several of the larger chains now offer veggie burgers on their menus and also offer fresh salads (simply ask for yours without chicken). If you know the secret password, you can get vegetarian sandwiches at McDonald's and Burger King; request a Big Mac without meat, and they'll be happy to comply. Ask for a veggie burger at Burger King, and you'll get tomato, lettuce, cheese (if you're ovo-lacto), and condiments on a bun.

Some chains, like Wendy's and Arby's, offer baked potatoes and lunchtime salad bars. And Taco Bell is a surprisingly good option for vegetarians; they use only vegetable oil in their cooking, even in their refried beans, and have a number of menu items that are good for ovo-lactos. Other chains have pita sandwiches and breakfast items like French toast sticks and scrambled eggs.

If you have concerns about what's in the food provided by your local fast-food purveyors, check out the nutritional information on the company's Web site. You might be surprised to learn that those French toast sticks are made without eggs or milk, and that McDonald's chocolate chip cookies are vegan. It pays, however, to check in occasionally and make sure menu items still contain the same ingredients, because if the company changes suppliers, the formulation may change too. The French fries at most fast-food restaurants are vegetarian, since they've pretty much all switched to 100 percent vegetable oil in response to public demand.

For your heartiest fast-food meal, look for restaurants that offer both salad bars and baked potatoes; not only is that a great meal combination, you can use salad bar toppings to customize your baked potato in whichever way you like.

Healthy Lunches at School or Work

If your school or workplace has a cafeteria, you may be in luck and they may offer vegetarian options. Institutional cooking is increasingly becoming health-conscious.

The option offering the most control for vegetarian children and teens is to brown-bag it and make them take their own lunch to school. If you're packing your own (or your kids') lunches, make sure to offer the same variety that you'd demand for yourself. Good lunch items include peanut butter or almond butter on whole wheat bread, carrot or celery stick with hummus spread, containers of fruit, pudding, or yogurt, Baggies of dried fruits and nuts, cartons of rice milk, string cheese, and protein bars.

Most schools send home schedules of what meals are planned for the week, so you can figure out ahead of time what hot meals can be eaten in the cafeteria and what days lunch should be brought from home. Sometimes, the ideal option might be to eat some of the cafeteria meal, like macaroni and cheese, and supplement it with fresh fruit, whole-grain crackers, and rice milk from home.

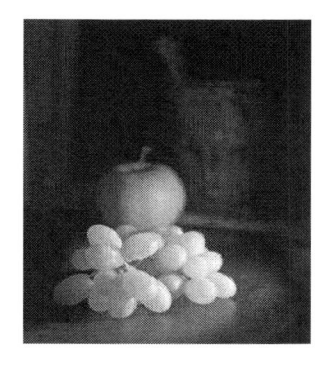

If you're a college student, you'll probably find that your food options include vegetarian meals; college is a time of experimentation, and most universities bend over backward to accommodate vegetarians (who are probably quite vocal about their needs). They also have bigger budgets and don't have to comply with the same food service restrictions as public schools, so you'll find a much wider range of healthy meal alternatives.

If you work for a big company, you may have a company cafeteria at your disposal. That may be great as they may have a salad bar or be vegetarian-friendly in their menu options. But there are equal chances of its being a grease pit that only offers greasy burgers and soggy fries.

It all depends on who's doing the cooking. Some company cafeterias have their own in-house chefs, in which case you can request that they provide some vegetarian menu items or even make you something special. Other companies contract out their food service, and it's made off-site.

The same strategies that apply to dealing with public school cafeterias can be used with your workplace cafeteria. If they offer a weekly menu, you can plan which days you'll eat in the cafeteria and when you'll bring your own lunch or eat out. You can also bring your own food and buy a couple of things in the cafeteria. One great advantage to being an adult employee is that, if you're dissatisfied with the vegetarian options in your company's cafeteria, you can meet with whoever coordinates the food service and ask if they can provide ovo-lacto or vegan options on a regular basis.

Restaurant Dining With Style

No matter how well you plan ahead, there will be times when you're in a restaurant and there's almost nothing on the menu that fits your vegetarian needs. That doesn't mean you should throw a hissy fit and pout; it means that you need to get a little creative.

Scan the menu, and look at what they offer. By examining their menu items, you can figure out what ingredients they use most frequently and ask for something combining those that they have on hand. If they offer spaghetti or fettuccine and steamed vegetables as a side dish, you can ask your server if the chef could put together a vegetarian pasta dish for you. If you're really stuck, you can make a meal of bread and salad, or ask for a baked potato.

But before you give up and make a meal of side dishes, ask your server nicely if the chef can accommodate a strict vegetarian. Odds are, they'll say yes. Then nicely tell them what you can and can't eat. Make sure you specify that you don't want any animal products, and let them know if that includes fish, cheese, eggs, or milk (surprisingly, even some chefs don't know what qualifies as vegetarian cuisine). If it turns out that they can't, thank your server for trying—after all, it's not their fault—and make do with what's available.

It pays, however, to understand a little bit about how the restaurant business operates. The waitstaff and cooks at diners and family-style restaurants will be less flexible when it comes to accommodating your off-menu requests. This isn't because they care less about their customers; it's because they are, due to the nature of their establishment, less flexible and creative. Ninety-nine percent of the customers who eat in such restaurants order straight off the menu, sometimes asking for simple adjustments like no butter on the toast or a side of sour cream. The waitstaff is accustomed to taking orders and getting food out fast, and the line cooks have mastered the standard menu items and rarely offer off-the-menu specials. Most of the time, the staff members at family restaurants simply don't know how to accommodate special dietary requests because they don't get those requests very often.

Fine dining establishments and neighborhood restaurants, though, are almost always better at handling special requests. The chefs are used to improvising and creating new menu items based on fresh local ingredients. The staff knows that customers need to be catered to so they'll keep coming back; the big chain restaurants care less about cultivating regulars because they know they'll still get lots of business no matter what.

Another advantage to eating in better restaurants is that, if you know in advance you'll be dining there, you can call ahead and let them know that there will be a vegetarian in your party. If you have a chance to look at their menu ahead of time, great; many restaurants now have their menus on the Web sites. But you can also call the day before, ask to speak to the manager or the chef, and specify that you'll be coming in at a certain time and tell them what your needs are. Don't just say, "I'm a vegetarian." Tell them that you don't eat any animal flesh (or eggs, cheese, and whatever your restrictions are), and you can even ask them if they can make sure your food isn't flavored with chicken or beef broth. For best results, don't dictate to them what you need; tell them politely, and ask for recommendations. If you're talking to the chef, he may come up with something terrific that isn't on the regular menu because it wouldn't normally sell well to their omnivorous clientele.

Even if something on the menu looks like it's probably a good choice, don't be shy about asking how the dish is prepared. It pays to know what certain cooking terms mean. "Au gratin" usually means that it's topped with cheese, and "scalloped" potatoes are made with a cream sauce. It's better for you, your server, and the chef if you make sure that you can eat something before you order it, rather than sending it back after it's been prepared because it turns out to contain ingredients you can't eat.

Also—remember those foods that often contain animal products like Caesar salad dressing, piecrusts, and tortillas. In restaurants, you'll also find that vegetables are sautéed in butter, spinach salad comes with bacon bits, split pea soup contains bits of ham, and potato salad has hard-cooked eggs. So ask your server about these things before you order, and then tip them accordingly for going the extra mile to make sure you get what you want!

CHAPTER 10

Balancing the Scales
Losing Weight while on a Vegetarian Diet

Americans spend over $30 billion each year on weight control products, programs, gym memberships, and gizmos. And yet, 25 percent of Americans are overweight, with about half of the women on weight-loss diets. The industries that make Americans fat, slim them down, and then fatten them up again— from the supersized fast-food corporations to the systems that are really just packaged food purveyors—get rich by advising people to eat irresponsibly. They're abetted by government agencies like the FDA and the USDA, which still promote their meat and carbohydrate-heavy food pyramid while chiding everyone for getting fat.

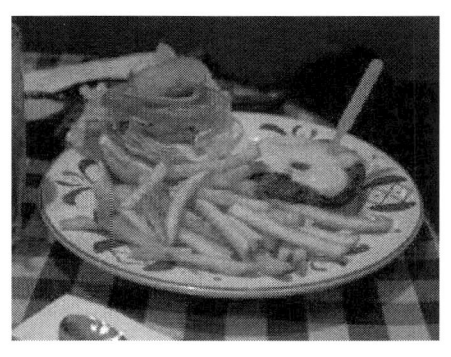

The diet industry rakes in the enormous profits that it does for one simple, yet ingenious, reason: the diets they promote don't work. Whether you try meal replacement shakes, prepackaged microwave meals, appetite suppressing pills, or the elimination of one major nutrient category (usually fats or carbohydrates), you'll find that all of these diets have one thing in common: while they're designed to take off weight in the short term, they aren't a diet plan that you can adapt for the rest of your life. Sooner or later (usually as soon as about half the weight you wanted to lose has melted away), you go back to eating real food instead of shakes, pills, bars, or boxed dinners, and the weight all comes back. Then you pronounce that diet a failure and jump on a different one!

This merry-go-round makes the diet industry very happy, and they're thrilled when a new fad comes along that they can exploit. When it was diet shakes, a hundred companies made diet shakes. When the boxed-meal diets became popular, five more programs opened franchises. The same company that was making low-fat meal replacement bars five years ago also turned out low-carb bars when the Atkins diet was all the rage and then switched back to making low-fat bars as soon as the fad started to fade. If the next big fad turns out to be an all-fish diet, you can bet those same companies will be manufacturing Cod Munchies and Halibut Delight Cookies.

The secret to successful weight control—or the secret that the diet industry doesn't want you to figure out—is eating a moderate amount of a variety of nutrient-rich foods. Because if you're eating whole foods, there's nothing for them to sell you! And the ideal weight control diet is a vegetarian diet. Vegetarians are, overall, thinner than nonvegetarians, despite eating everything that the diet programs forbid.

Rethinking the Concept of Dieting

Going by conventional wisdom, it doesn't make sense that vegetarians can be slender when they eat potatoes, pasta, bread, beans, and rice. This, in fact, is the first clue that the conventional wisdom is wrong. Popular fad diets insist that starchy foods will pack on the pounds and insist that you limit carbohydrates to a small green salad and maybe one piece of fresh fruit each day. But vegetarianism is a naturally slenderizing diet and one that makes sense when you understand just how it fuels the body.

If you want to lose weight permanently and stay off fad diets forever, the first step is to jettison everything that the diet gurus have told you. Starvation diets—and really, that's what all fad diets are—don't keep weight off in the long term.

A realistic diet is one that contains whole, healthful foods and doesn't involve buying special products and supplements. You don't need to count calories or points or talk to a diet counselor every week. You just need to change the way you eat and replace old bad habits with new good ones.

Face it. If you're fat, it's because of the way you eat. And the only way to change that is to revamp your diet and have some patience. It took a long time to gain all that weight, and it's going to take a long time to get it off. If you want to lose weight and keep it off for the rest of your life, you have to find a way of eating that you can live with even after you're at your ideal weight. There are no quick fixes—not if you want permanent results.

It's a Lifestyle, Not a Diet

Throughout this book, we've referred to the vegetarian diet, with the word "diet" being used in its original sense—your overall system of nourishing yourself. As a vegetarian, you're changing your diet but you're not on a diet, which is a significant difference. But they both systems focus on one thing: calories. A healthy diet, however, doesn't involve counting calories and withholding food so the body starves. A healthy diet allows the body ample calories so that every one of its functions like a well-oiled machine, burning fuel as it hums along.

Calories are units of energy, like the gallons of gas you use to fuel your car. You consume calories when you eat, and your body burns the energy to fuel all the things that it needs to do. Whether you're running around the block or sitting on the couch watching television, your body is burning energy to keep your heart pumping, your lungs and kidneys functioning, your brain working, and your muscles contracting.

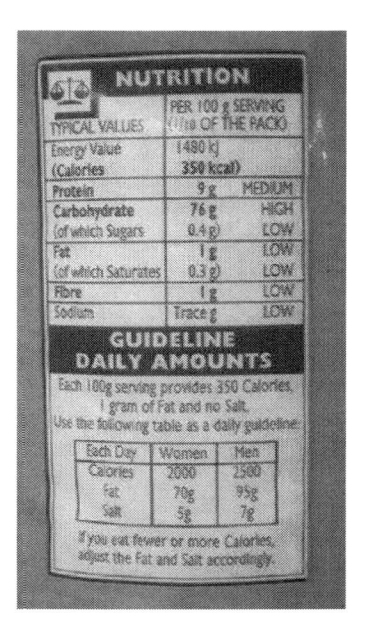

The pace at which your body burns calories when at rest is called "basal metabolism." That's when you burn most of your calories, actually—during sleeping or just sitting around. You burn them at a faster rate when you're exercising and digesting food, but your basal metabolism determines how many calories you need to function, with the excess being stored as fat.

As you're no doubt aware, some people have faster metabolisms, while others have sluggish ones. Men usually have higher metabolisms than women because they have more muscle mass. People who exercise regularly can raise their metabolism, so they burn more calories even when they're at rest.

Whatever the speed of the metabolism, though, it's fuel is the calories. Foods that have a lot of calories are loaded with fuel from protein, carbohydrates, and fat. If you eat the same amount of calories that you need to fuel your body, you can maintain your ideal weight. Take in more calories than you burn, and you store the excess calories as fat. Weight loss occurs when you consume less calories than your body needs to burn for energy. When it needs fuel, the body turns to the stored fat and breaks it down into usable energy. You can make this happen on purpose by either exercising and burning a lot of calories, or by eating less.

As you'll remember from previous chapters, our bodies are amazing evolutionary machines and are designed to survive when there's no food available. When you drastically cut back on the calories you eat, your body thinks that you're in danger of starving and slows down your metabolism so that you aren't burning as much energy. This is why most people on calorie-restrictive diets lose quickly at first and then slow down to a crawl—or plateau, at which point they aren't losing at all even when they're hardly eating anything at all.

Many people believe that exercise is the answer to boosting metabolism, but it's only part of the equation. If you're eating a very low-calorie diet and exercising a lot, your body is still going to believe that it's starving, so the weight loss will be very, very slow. That's not to say that exercise isn't important; maintaining strong muscles helps you stay active and keeps you burning fat, no matter how slowly. But you still need to eat a moderate number of calories to keep your metabolism functioning well so that your body doesn't go into starvation mode, and finding the right balance can be frustrating to dieters who want to see big results quickly.

Not All Calories Are Alike

Despite all the advances in nutritional science, most people still believe that losing weight is merely a matter of eating less food. Even a lot of doctors believe it, and they, of all people, ought to know better! But in truth, many overweight people eat less than thin people, the only difference being they just eat the wrong things.

Of the three main categories of nutrients—protein, carbohydrates, and fat—it's the fat that contains the most calories. Protein and carbohydrates contain four calories per gram; a gram of fat, on the other hand, contains nine calories. So while fat is an important nutrient for many reasons—like keeping your hormones regulated, your skin and hair healthy, and giving you a feeling of satiety when you eat—it also provides over twice as many calories as protein and carbs. And what foods are the highest in fat? Animal foods.

Plant foods, though, are rich in complex carbohydrates, so you can eat more food while ingesting less calories; this will make you feel fuller and more satisfied. Naturally, you can gain weight while eating carbohydrate-rich foods; remember that excess calories, no matter what their source, are stored as body fat. But studies have shown that, while people eating low-fat, high-carb diets consume more than people on higher fat diets, they're taking in less calories! In a study at Cornell University, people choosing a diet restricting their fat intake of 20 to 25 percent of their calories ate more food than the subjects choosing a diet of 35 to 40 percent fat, but they never ingested as many calories as the high-fat group.

But there's more to the story than just calories. While doctors and nutritionalists have always advised that dieting is strictly a lower-your-calories endeavor, current research is revealing that it's far more complicated than that. The way the body uses the calories from protein, carbs, and fat varies depending on the source of those calories. The human body is designed to store energy from fats and proteins while it burns carbs for immediate energy. We're just not meant to store carbohydrates; for every one hundred calories that you eat, twenty-three are burned just converting the carbs to usable energy! The fat we eat is a double whammy; not only are there more calories per gram of fat, only three of every one hundred calories are burned during conversion, meaning that it's later to burn as energy and stored as excess body fat more easily.

The nature of carbohydrates is that they're the first type of energy that our body turns to, which makes it actually difficult to store carbs as fat. In a 1991 clinical study, only 2 percent of the calories eaten by subjects were converted into fat. So while calories are important, it's the fat calories that are best cut back on.

It's also possible to lose weight on a high-protein, low-fat diet, but there are reasons why that is a bad idea. For one thing, it isn't easy. The whole foods highest in protein are animal foods, so they're also high in fat. Perhaps you've tried one of these diets in the past and discovered that eating scrambled egg whites, skinless chicken breasts, and dry, broiled fish gets boring very quickly. But another reason to steer clear of high-protein diets is the difficulty, discussed in an earlier chapter, that your body has processing protein. Too much protein overtaxes your kidneys, and it builds calcium deposits in your bones and urinary tract. So the best overall weight-loss plan is one that gives you energy from healthy, complex carbohydrates derived from plant sources.

Natural, Plant-based Weight Control

By switching to vegetarianism, you've probably already noticed a boost in your health and may have already lost a few pounds without even trying. The standard vegetarian diet is naturally high in complex carbohydrates and low in fat; a vegan diet, with all the nutrients coming from plant foods, is the lowest in fat of all.

But it's still possible to eat too much fat. Nuts, seeds, avocados, and olives are all high in fat. And as we've already mentioned, just being vegetarian doesn't guarantee that you're eating a healthy diet if you're constantly munching on fries, chips, and cookies. So while you've got a good head start on weight control by becoming vegetarian, you still need to give your diet some thought.

We'll discuss meal planning and give you some great recipes in the upcoming chapters, but for now, let's consider the basics of your vegetarian choices with an eye toward weight control.

Vegetables are, of course, the mainstay of your daily diet. Use fresh whenever possible, frozen if you have to, and stay away from canned vegetables (canned products usually contain a lot of sodium and, well, they just don't taste very good). Steam them and squeeze some lemon juice on them, or eat them with nonfat dressing. If you insist on sautéing them in fat, use olive oil.

Fruit can be fresh, frozen, or if necessary, canned (beware of sugary syrups, though). Fruit juice has more calories than whole fruit, and you're missing out on the fiber, so eat whole fruit whenever possible.

Grains should be processed as little as possible; go with whole-grain products for better texture, more fiber, and more nutrients. For breakfast, hot cereals are usually higher in fiber and lower in fat than cold cereals, and keep an eye on how much fat is in favorites like muffins, pancakes, snack crackers, and biscuits.

Legumes are excellent sources of high-protein, low-fat nutrition. Beans are loaded with nutrition, although, if you use canned beans, watch out for added salt. Veggie burgers and hot dogs are healthier options than their meat-based counterparts, but they can still add a hefty amount of fat to your diet if you rely on them too much. Read labels, and make processed foods a small part of your diet.

Nuts and seeds are good sources of important nutrients but contain up to 70 percent fat. While trying to lose weight, limit the amount of these to one serving each day. You can increase the amount when you're at the point of maintaining your weight—but still watch those portions!

Dairy products, remember, are derived from milk—a substance high in both fat and sugar that is meant to fatten up baby cows. If you're ovo-lacto, drink 1 percent or skim milk. Rice milk is tasty, and lower in calories than regular milk. Cheese is very high in fat and should only be used in very small amounts when trying to lose weight.

Fats must be used sparingly, if at all, when cooking on a weight-loss diet. Whenever possible, use olive oil, but eliminate fats by steaming, broiling, or baking foods instead of frying or sautéing. If you're eating a well-balanced diet, you're getting all the fat you need to keep your body healthy, so don't add more.

Skinny Vegetarianism

Carbohydrates have gotten a bad rap in recent years, but the biggest sin isn't how many carbs we eat—it's the manner in which we eat them. We dunk perfectly good potatoes in hot oil, or soak them in butter, or cover them with cream sauce. We spread an inch of butter on our whole-wheat rolls and cover our broccoli with cheese sauce. No wonder we're fat!

Transitioning to a plant-based diet is about thoughtful, healthy eating. That holds true for the way you prepare the food that you eat, too. Many people think they don't like vegetables when, in fact, they rarely taste the vegetables they eat because they're drowning in a puddle of butter sauce. Give your food the same respect that you give your body, and enjoy it without disguising it with a high-fat coating.

Choose healthy substitutions when snacking. Instead of reaching for greasy potato chips or an order of fries, grab a handful of fat-free pretzels or popcorn. Dunk celery and carrots into hummus, salsa, or black bean dip instead of guacamole.

Lower the fat in your baked foods. Almost any cookie, cake, or muffin recipe can be made with less fat, and there are recipes for low-fat baked foods using applesauce or mashed bananas as a fat substitute. Whole-wheat pastry flour has less gluten than all-purpose flour and will make an even tender product when you're cutting down on fat.

Learn to love the spud. As the basis for a meal, it's hard to beat a baked potato. With less than a gram of fat, just ninety-five calories, and loads of vitamins, it's an almost perfect natural food. But once you've piled on butter, sour cream, and cheese, it's a nutritional nightmare. There are lots of things you can use to top your potato. Vegetarian chili, vegetable curry, baked beans, and steamed vegetables are all great potato toppers, low in fat, and loaded with vitamins and minerals.

Add flavor, not fat. Think about the flavors in the foods you're cooking and consider ways to enhance them without added fat. Sauté vegetables in dry wine, use fresh herbs and garlic, and freshen up vegetables with lemon juice.

Avoid the dairy trap. Ovo-lacto-vegetarians often make the mistake of leaning too much on eggs, cheese, milk, yogurt, and other dairy products when they first start out, and these foods are all rich in fat. Go easy on the cheese, drink skim milk, and limit eggs to just two or three meals per week.

Snacking While Trying to Lose Weight

Not everything that is labeled vegetarian is low in fat. Eat the following in moderation when trying to lose weight:

- Almond butter
- Avocados
- Coconut
- Falafel
- French fries
- Hummus
- Olives
- Packaged vegetarian meals
- Peanut butter
- Potato chips
- Tahini

There are lots of snacks that fit into your vegetarian eating plan and are great for weight loss diets too. When you want something between meals, reach for one of these:

- Bagels
- Bean soup
- Fresh fruit
- Fresh vegetables
- High-fiber cereal
- Nonfat crackers
- Pita bread or chips
- Potatoes–baked, broiled, or grilled
- Pretzels
- Rice cakes
- Whole-grain rolls and muffins

Breaking the Diet Cycle

Every day, every week Americans struggle to stick to their diet. They monitor what they eat and how many calories they burn in a constant effort to achieve a certain weight. Let's face it. Diets are unproductive, unfulfilling, and restrictive. As soon the diet ends, they ultimately put the weight back on because they never addressed the core issue, and the cycle of dieting repeats itself.

Who wants to live like that?

According to *The Food Revolution* by John Robbins, the relative sliminess of vegetarians was made abundantly clear in a chapter discussing weight loss. An experienced doctor who performed liposuction procedures told Robbins that more than one thousand liposuctions were performed on any given day, every day of the week. That's a lot of fat! But what's even more astounding is that the doctor also told Robbins that, out of all the operations he had performed, he couldn't remember operating on a vegetarian—ever. What does that tell you?

Our society has a tendency to focus on the outside of the body instead of on the inside. But being beautiful starts on the inside and permeates outward, and that starts by paying attention to what you eat and how you eat. There is no fad diet out there that will work over a long period of time, and quick-fix diets always end in disaster when you gain even more weight back than you lost in the first place. Do yourself a favor and break the diet cycle. It doesn't matter how many weight-loss programs you sign up for or how many diet books you read; becoming a vegetarian is the best thing you can do to break the cycle.

Healthy Doesn't Always Mean Skinny

Body types are often dictated by genes. Some people are naturally small and slender, others are destined to be thicker of build. If you're a woman, this may mean that you're a little heavier in the thighs or that your general build is athletic, even if you'd prefer to be lithe. The truth is, there's little you can do about that. And you may have a genetic tendency to be overweight, which is passed on from your parents and grandparents.

Eating well and exercising will get you into better shape no matter what your body type, but you may never be truly thin without starving yourself. If you're fixated on a specific number on the scale but you can't reach it no matter how much you work out and how little you eat, it may be time to accept that you're where you're supposed to be.

That's not to say that, if you have either a moderate amount of weight to lose or a lot, you should give up and accept your overweight state. If you come from a family of overweight people, genetics is only a small part of the picture. Do you have the same eating habits as your parents? Were they sedentary, spending all of their free time on the couch and eating fatty snack foods?

By developing healthy eating habits now, and exercising, you can break the cycle and become the best you that you can be. There are no guarantees where weight loss is concerned, but a low-fat vegetarian diet can get you to where you'll be healthier and happier, whatever your weight.

CHAPTER 11

Exercising the Mind, Body, and Spirit—Vegetarian Style

Everyone knows the importance of exercise. Humans were not made to live sedentary lives. We were made to get up and move, which is precisely why we have legs. The mind, body, and spirit are all connected, and when they are healthy, they work in per.fect harmony with one another. One way of aligning these three key elements is through physical activity. Whether it's taking a nice walk outside, participating in an athletic event, or going to the gym, you will easily see the benefits of being active. When you pair exercise with a nutritional vegetarian diet, you've got the recipe for a healthier life, longevity, and a positive attitude combined with an overall sense of well-being.

Get Moving–One Step at a Time

Many people steer clear of exercise because they aren't sure what they should be doing. They don't know what kind of activity to do. It can be confusing because there are differing opinions circulating out there. Some fitness gurus emphasize rigorous routines that can easily turn away an exercise beginner. Others jump on certain bandwagons, like kickboxing or some other Hollywood fitness trend. The truth is that the activity itself does not matter; what matters most is that you stay active. And this can be accomplished quite easily. If you enjoy team sports, join a local softball league or find a sport that you like to play. These leagues are normally very inclusive, and games are played once or twice a week so that you can fit them into your schedule. If you own a dog, take him or her for walks before or after work. Pay a visit to the park over the weekend and play with your dog for a little while. You'll be surprised at how much activity you can get from simply playing with your pet!

If you are someone who doesn't like to exercise alone, recruit a friend. Go for walks together, or schedule time to go to the gym together. When you have a caring confidant there to listen to you and support you, sticking to an exercise regiment is that much easier. Joining a gym is also a great way to meet people and make friends. Most gyms offer training sessions, fun exercise classes, and numerous health-awareness programs. For $30 a month or less, you can gain a wealth of knowledge about the benefits of exercise. That's not a lot to pay for something that will increase your overall health.

There are many ways to be active. But it all starts with the first step. Once you take the first step, the second and third will follow. If you don't believe me, try get up off of the couch and go for a walk instead of watching television after work. Even if you can only walk around the block, you'll feel a new sense of aliveness within you. And the next day, you'll be able to walk a step further. A woman, who was recently interviewed on *Good Morning America* because she lost over 250 pounds, said that it all started with the first step. One day, she just got up and started walking. At first, she could only walk a few minutes before stopping. Now, she walks three to four miles a day!

Exercising on a Vegetarian Diet

Just because you are eating less meat and a lot more vegetables and fruit doesn't mean you don't have to exercise. Since you will be eating a lot more carbohydrates, you need to burn up the excess energy. Exercising will also help get rid of any toxins that may be lurking in your body through sweat. Active vegetarians who limit their carbohydrate intake will definitely begin to feel sluggish. Just make sure that you are eating the right kinds of carbohydrates.

Good selections of carbohydrates include:

> Pasta
> Beans
> Rice

Potatoes
Lentils
Breads
Vegetables
Fruits
Grains (cereal)
Rice milk

Some beginner vegetarians who are active worry that they won't be getting enough nutrients to keep up their exercise regime. But the increase in nutritional needs for noncompetitive athletes or people who exercise four or five days per week is really quite small. It's mostly professional athletes and Olympic athletes who need to worry about their diet and make sure that they are getting all the nutrients they need to stay competitive. However, if you are active on a regular basis, you need to make sure that you are getting plenty of carbohydrates to burn, with an adequate amount of protein and fats. Getting enough calories and carbohydrates in your daily routine will help circulate the protein in your body directly to your muscles for growth and repair.

Foods that can easily boost your protein intake include:

A large bowl of hot cereal (whole grain), like oatmeal, with rice or hemp milk
A bagel with peanut butter
Hummus and carrots
A baked potato
Yogurt with granola
A protein fruit smoothie made with rice milk
A bowl of vegetarian chili
Bean burritos
Pasta made with pesto

What you should limit is your intake of saturated fats. If you are having some trouble getting enough calories into your vegetarian diet, it's okay to add a little saturated fat now and then. It doesn't take a lot of saturated fat to boost your calorie count. Just be careful not to eat too much of it!

Top Ten Reasons Why Exercising Is Good for You

I have given you some extremely good reasons to exercise so far, but if you need a little more convincing here are some points you can consider:

1. Exercise gives you brainpower. Not only does consistent exercise help improve your body, but it also helps improve your brain by increasing the levels of serotonin, which directly leads to mental clarity. Individuals who exercise are more productive throughout the day than those individuals who don't.

2. Say good-bye to stress. It is a proven fact that exercise reduces stress because it increases the endorphins in your body, which directly affect your mood and help keep stress and depression at bay. Watch how the situations and relationships in your life begin to improve simply by exercising a few times every week.

3. You'll be more energized. You probably think that by exercising you will be more tired throughout the day. That isn't the case at all! Actually, when you exercise on a regular basis, you will feel more energized. Work out for thirty minutes in the morning, and see what happens. The endorphins you release will keep you focused and attentive for the duration of the day! When you improve your strength and stamina, you will be able to accomplish more tasks throughout the day without feeling exhausted when you get home.

4. Finding time to exercise is actually easy. Many people use the excuse that there isn't enough time to avoid exercising. Think about how many hours per day you spend watching television. By trimming off just thirty minutes from that time, you now have thirty minutes to exercise instead. In fact, you'd be surprised at how easy it is to find ten minutes to spare here or twenty minutes to spare there.

5. Exercising makes you socially active. Whether you exercise with a partner, a sibling, or a friend, your relationship with that person will most likely improve. Exercise is more fun when you have someone to do it with. Instead of two ships passing in the night, go for a walk with your spouse after work. You will add another level of intimacy and communication to your relationship. By joining a gym or league sport, you also have the opportunity to meet new friends and form newer and more positive relationships.

6. You'll maintain a healthier body. Studies have shown that frequent exercising is essential in preventing the development of major diseases such as heart disease, stroke, high blood pressure, and diabetes. It can even help ward off common colds by boosting your immune system.

7. You'll have a healthier heart. Your heart is the command center of your body. By exercising, you can create a stronger heart, which will help your cardiovascular system to function more effectively. Watch how your level of fatigue decreases simply by exercising for a few days. The results speak for themselves.

8. You can eat more of the foods you like. Even vegetarians like to indulge in sweets now and then. When you exercise, you can enjoy these temptation foods without feeling guilty because you are burning more calories on a regular basis.

9. You'll love the way you look. Looks aren't everything, but when you exercise, you will definitely look and feel better. Your clothes will also fit your body better because of the lean muscle you are building. You may notice that your arms and stomach look a bit firmer, and I guarantee you'll like what you see.

10. It's more than just losing a few pounds. Weight loss is a wonderful benefit of exercising, but it's not the only benefit. When you look and feel better, and are more productive and healthy, everything in your life falls in sync. The overall enhancement of health is the real goal of exercising. And losing a few pounds here or there is just an added bonus!

CHAPTER 12

The Meatless Kitchen
Buying Food and Planning Menus

Ever visit the kitchen of an avid cook? It's organized, clean, well-stocked, and ready for whatever creative menus strike their fancy. Eating well isn't just about the food you eat; it's also about having the tools you need to make great meals. Organization, planning, and cleanliness will make cooking in your kitchen a pleasure rather than a chore.

Managing Your Workspace

Whether you enjoy spending hours in the kitchen chopping, stirring, and mixing (or you just want to get in and get out quickly), it pays to make your kitchen into a place that you enjoy spending time. That means that the kitchen will be clean, organized, and having the equipment you need to do the job.

Step one to organizing your kitchen is to go through your cupboards and get rid of all the accumulated stuff that you don't have any use for. That means broken appliances (and the ones you got as Christmas gifts that you've never used), old paper plates from kids' birthday parties, half-empty bottles of hot sauce that you've had for six years, and those empty jars that are gathering dust on the top shelf. If you're not going to use it, toss it out, give it away, or sell it online; just get it out of your workspace.

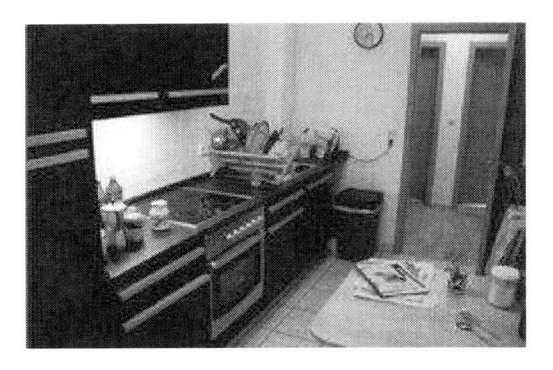

Take your kitchen, one section at a time, and clean off the shelves. Wipe them clean with a cleanser, maybe lay down some fresh shelf paper. Do the same with your drawers. You don't have to do it all in one night; take it a little at a time with the goal of getting all your shelves and drawers sparkling clean. Scrub down the stove, and clean your refrigerator inside and outside. Throw away the food that's gone bad or that has been sitting there for ages because you'll never eat it. Toss out any foods in your cupboards that are going to waste too.

Right now, there's probably a haphazard plan, at best, to the way your kitchen is arranged. Your pots and pans are a jumble in one cupboard, your wooden spoons, spatulas, and knives all tossed in the same drawer, and your cookie sheets are leaning against the wall. The dry goods on your shelves—cereal, pasta, and the like—are probably left on the shelves with no regard for organization. It takes time to find things when you want to use them, and there's an attitude of disrespect when you treat your food and your tools this way. Your new lifestyle is about healthy habits, right? So develop good organizational habits too!

Start by organizing things by type. Put all of your fats, oils, salad dressings, and condiments together. Pasta, rice, and other uncooked grains should be together too. Think of how they're stocked when you go to the grocery store—there's an intuitive design behind the methods that grocers stock their goods. The same rules make sense in your kitchen too. Organize your spices, as well. You don't have to go as far as to alphabetize them, but you can find an organizational system that works for you, like putting the things you use the most in the front, or separating the herbs and the spices.

Handling the Hardware

There are tools that you'll need to cook with, but not as many as you might think—and possibly not even as many as you already own. If your countertop is cluttered with a coffeemaker, a mixer, a blender, a toaster, an oven, and a microwave, ask yourself how often you use these items. Do they need to be there all the time? If you rarely bake, store the mixer under a counter until you need it. Ditto to the blender. If you only make a pot of coffee on the weekend, think about storing it out of sight during the week. This will give you more space to work and make your kitchen look less cluttered.

If you don't cook much, you may find yourself lacking some basic kitchen essentials. Most can be purchased inexpensively at stores like Target or Wal-Mart, but you can find a lot of them for almost nothing at thrift stores. The basics for any home kitchen include:

> Measuring cups and spoons
> Bowls in various sizes for mixing and serving
> Wooden spoons
> Rubber spatulas
> Whisks
> Baking pans and cookie sheets
> Pots and pans in assorted sizes
> Good, sharp knives—a paring knife, a chef's knife, and a serrated bread knife
>
> Bigger items that you'll probably want include:
>
> A mixer, either countertop style or handheld
> Heavy-duty blender
> Food processor
> Slow cooker (usually called a crock pot)
> Rice cooker

The Vegetarian Pantry

Grains are versatile, have a long shelf life, and are inexpensive; they are therefore the perfect pantry staple. Store them in airtight containers in a cool, dry place away from sunlight, and they're good for months. If you have the space in your fridge or freezer, they'll last longer if you store them there; just make sure they're well sealed to keep out moisture.

Most of the grain products you'll want to stock are already familiar to you: whole wheat breads and pancakes mixes, breakfast cereals, pasta, tortillas, and bulk grains like rice and oats. But now that you're going to be eating a diet rich in plant foods, this is a good time to learn about new grains you've never tried, as well as educate yourself about your old favorites.

Barley is a grain that's gone out of fashion, although it's been a staple food for generations. It's great in vegetable soups, giving them a nutty taste and delightfully chewy texture. You can buy it as a whole grain at your health food store. Barley is loaded with nutrients but takes a long time to cook. Pearl barley has the tough outer bran shell removed, so it offers less fiber—but it cooks faster and is still delicious. Add it to your soups, stews, and vegetarian chili; use it in casseroles and sauté it with veggies.

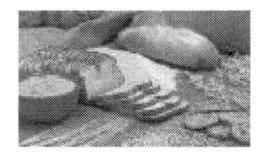

Cornmeal is dried, ground corn that, if you've ever used it at all, you've probably only used to make corn bread. Now is the time to introduce yourself to polenta, a delicious, savory Italian porridge that can be eaten hot or cold (look for a recipe in chapter 13). Add it to your homemade breads for great flavor and texture.

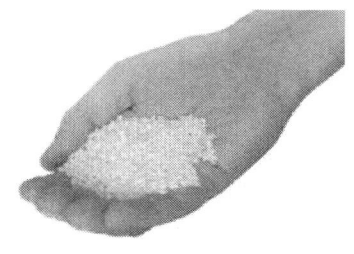

Rice is an old standby, but there's more to it than the basic white stuff you get with your Chinese food. A good rule of thumb to remember is that the shorter the grain, the starchier the rice. Long-grain rice stays fluffy with separate grains, and it's the choice for pilaf. Medium-grain rice—the kind found in most American kitchens—is soft and fluffy when cooked but gets stickier as it cools. Short-grain rice is the starchy, thick, gluey kind served with Asian and Indian cuisine. There's a world of different rice that is available in these three types. Arborio is a very short-grained rice used to make risotto (although any short-grain white rice can be used); basmati is an aromatic long-grain rice, available as either brown or white rice, that's imported from India and Pakistan (although it's also grown commercially in Texas); japonica rice is a very sticky Japanese rice; brown rice is whole kernels of rice with the nutty outer shell still intact; and jasmine rice is a yummy, highly aromatic long grain rice that's great for cold salads, as it stays fluffy long after cooking. There's also wild rice, which isn't actually rice at all; it's a grass seed that grows wild in the Midwest and is usually combined with different kinds of rice because it is somewhat expensive.

Quinoa is an ancient food staple that dates back to the Incas. It's great in cold salads or when seasoned with herbs and served with potatoes.

Buckwheat, when toasted, is called kasha, and it has a strong flavor. Untoasted, it's decidedly mellower, and a welcome addition to pancakes and breads.

Legumes—beans, mostly—are also a great food to always have in stock, either dry or canned. Dried beans have a long shelf life, and they're both versatile and nutritious. Rinse canned beans well before you use them to remove the excess sodium. Like grains, there are many, many different types of beans, good in all sorts of different dishes. And they're inexpensive, so you can experiment without breaking your budget.

Kidney beans are the traditional white or red beans used in soups, stews, and chili. You should always have these on hand, because you'll find hundreds of uses for them.

Navy beans are the small, pale beans used in that old favorite, navy bean soup. You can also use them to make your own vegetarian baked beans.

Split peas come in green or yellow varieties, and are some of the fastest-cooking varieties of the legumes. Use them to make old-fashioned split pea soup, or branch out and make some of the many delicious Indian dishes that use them.

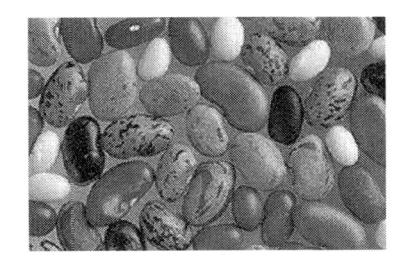

Black-eyed peas aren't peas at all but beans that were brought to America from Africa by slaves; they are a staple in Southern cooking. Unlike most beans, these don't need to be soaked first; they cook quickly and are great in spicy main dishes.

Black turtle beans hail from Central America and the Caribbean, and they're delicious in spicy dishes like chili and burritos.

Cannellini beans are small white beans used in Italian soups and other dishes. Use them in soups or salads.

Chickpeas are also called garbanzo beans and are a common ingredient in Mediterranean cuisine. These are the soft, round, light brown beans you find at salad bars. Learn to use them in cooking and you can make your own hummus, tahini, and vegetarian curries.

Great northern beans are big, white beans with a very subtle flavor. They're great for soups.

Lima beans, also called butter beans, are wide, green soft beans with a delicious flavor. Eat them raw with just a little salt and pepper, or use them to make succotash, a traditional Southern dish.

Lentils are one of the oldest foods known to man and are a staple of Indian and Middle Eastern cuisine.

Soybeans are high in protein and low in fat, and can be included in any dish that traditionally uses beans. They take a while to cook and have a subtle flavor. Use them in baked beans, spicy soups, and ethnic dishes. (Be careful if you want to consume soy; there are warnings about soy throughout this book.)

A Well-rounded Larder

Stocking a variety of nuts, vegetables, and condiments can help you keep your diet interesting and inspire you in your cooking. In no particular order, here are foods that ought to be on every vegetarian's shopping list:

Nuts, seeds, and nut butters, like cashews, walnuts, hazelnuts, pecans, pine nuts, sesame seeds, sunflower seeds, almond butter, cashew butter, and peanut butter. Nut butters should be stored in a cool, dry place; nuts and seeds can be frozen for longer shelf life.

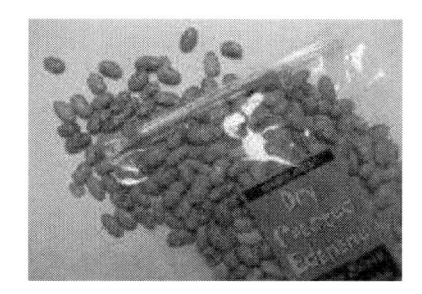

Tofu is a key ingredient in some vegetarian diets. There are some concerns about soy products in general because of mixed reviews and numerous studies evaluating the pros and cons. We will address those concerns in chapter 14 so that you can make an informed decision about eating soy and soy products like tofu. Tofu comes in different textures. It is extra-firm for stir-fries and acts as an egg substitute in egg salad recipes; soft tofu can be used as a substitute for sour cream, or it can be combined with chocolate for a protein-rich, dairy-free pudding. Tempeh is fermented tofu, and it has a mushroomlike flavor. Textured vegetable protein, or TVP, is a dried soy product that, when reconstituted, resembles ground beef. It can be used in soups, stir-fries, burritos, and any other recipe in which you'd use ground beef.

Dried fruit like apples, apricots, raisins, dates, figs, and banana chips are good for a quick snack or to combat low blood sugar. But they should be eaten in moderation, as they're very high in calories.

Condiments and other ingredients like barbecue sauce, ketchup, mustard and egg-free mayonnaise are obvious pantry staples. But also consider stocking nutritional yeast, an inactive, vitamin-rich yeast that can be mixed with grains or sprinkled on popcorn; canned coconut milk for making curries; marinated artichokes for salads and casseroles; hoisin sauce, a sweet Chinese condiment made from soybeans; fresh garlic and ginger; curry paste; olives and pickles; dehydrated sun-dried tomatoes, wasabi, a very hot powder made from a Japanese radish; vegetarian Worcestershire sauce; and tamari, traditional, fermented soy sauce.

Vinegars are good for cooking and homemade salad dressings; they include apple cider vinegar, balsamic vinegar, raspberry vinegar, red and white wine vinegars, and herb-infused vinegars.

Processed grains are necessary for baking. All-purpose whole-wheat flour is the most obvious, but you'll need higher-gluten bread flour for making bread and low-gluten pastry flour for baking muffins, cakes, and cookies. Other grains that are good for breads are rye flour, oat flour, wheat bran, and wheat germ.

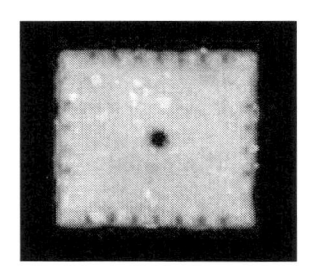

Cereals, bread, and crackers are as basic to a vegetarian diet as they are to an omnivorous one. You'll want whole-grain bread and rolls, oatmeal (good for hot cereal and for cookies), ready-to-eat whole-grain cereals, graham crackers, pita bread, rice cakes, and whole-grain crackers.

Canned foods aren't ideal, but sometimes you need them to make a quick meal you can throw together in a flash. Keep on hand cans of beans, pumpkin, tomatoes (crushed, diced, or whole), tomato paste, and spaghetti sauce.

Beverages like coffee and tea are probably already on your shelves, and you should also try different rice milks, as well as almond milk.

Meat substitutes like veggie burgers and hot dogs should be a small part of your diet, but keep some in the freezer for fast meals.

Baking ingredients like baking soda and baking powder are standard kitchen fare, but also pick up arrowroot, a thickener that can be used in place of cornstarch and dairy-free egg substitutes.

Sweeteners should be used sparingly, but there are a few that offer slightly more nutrient value than refined white sugar (a product that many vegans reject because it's sometimes processed using animal products). Honey offers trace nutrients, but it can't be used by vegans; maple sugar has a characteristic maple flavor and is good on cereal or in baked foods; barley-malt syrup is extracted from roasted barley and is excellent in baked foods; *stevia* is a sweet herb whose dried, powdered leaves are made into a low-calorie sweetener that's three hundred times sweeter than sugar.

Herbs and spices are a given, and what you want to keep on your shelves depends on your menu plans. The basics are basil, bay leaves, oregano, rosemary, sage, tarragon, thyme, allspice, cardamom, cayenne, chili powder, cinnamon, cloves, coriander, cumin, garlic powder, ginger, nutmeg, paprika, and turmeric.

Planning Your Meals: Breakfast

You've heard your whole life that breakfast is the most important meal of the day, and it's true. After eight hours of sleep, you want to jump-start your brain and body with a carbohydrate-rich meal, and get your engine revving for the rest of the day. If you're not a fan of breakfast, this is a good time to make the meal a part of your new, healthy habits. And if you do enjoy an early-morning meal, you'll probably find that your vegetarian breakfast is your favorite meal of the day.

For traditionalists, you can easily modify basic fare to meet ovo-lacto or vegan needs. Vegetarian sausage or fake bacon is a fine substitute for the real thing, and a chickpea scramble offers the same protein boost as eggs. Round it out with whole-wheat pancakes and coffee, and all you need is the morning newspaper.

Breakfast doesn't need to involve cooking. A bowl of cereal, hot or cold, with hemp milk and a glass of juice is a balanced breakfast. A slice of toast with peanut butter and a piece of fruit is a quick meal, too. Many people prefer something simple and quick in the morning. Just because you've gone vegetarian doesn't mean that you have to turn every meal into a production!

Anything you like to eat can be breakfast. Leftover lasagna, a slice of cold pizza, or reheated Chinese food is as good for you in the morning as they are at night. Microwave a frozen vegetarian entrée, or have some lentil curry. It's up to you, so eat whatever you like best.

Have breakfast any time; the same eat-what-you-like rule applies at lunch or dinner. There's no rule that says you can't enjoy pancakes and vegetarian sausage for your evening meal.

Planning Your Meals: Lunch

Lunch is a great meal, because you can eat just about anything you want, from breakfast foods to sandwiches to soups and salads. Borrow ideas from other meals for your midday repast—waffles with fruit compote, or a bowl of chili and a whole-wheat muffin.

If you take your lunch to work or school, invest in a small, insulated lunch bag. Pop in a reusable freezer insert, and keep you cold stuff cold all day. Or freeze a bottle of water and place that in your bag; it'll be thawed in time for lunch and serve double duty by keeping your lunch chilled!

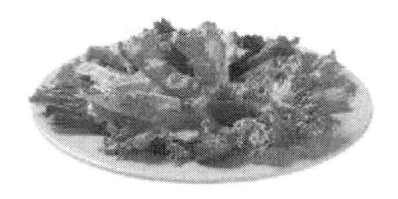

You remember how great those big salads that you bought in restaurants were? You can make your own fabulous salad to eat either at home or at work. You just need the right ingredients! Mixed greens, romaine, butter lettuce (or a combination) is your base. Add tomatoes, shredded soy-free cheese, sunflower seeds, sliced red pepper, or any other thing that sounds appealing. If you take it to work, put a serving of salad dressing in a separate container so your salad stays crisp until mealtime.

If you miss favorites like tuna or chicken salad, make vegetarian versions using tempeh or other meat alternatives. Load them into a pita pocket with some lettuce and tomatoes and you have a hearty meal.

If you forget to bring your lunch and know there won't be the time or the opportunity to get something on your work break, pick up something on the way to work. Most fast-food restaurants are open quite early in the morning, so stop in and get a bean burrito, big salad, or veggie burger during your morning commute. Stash it in you desk or the office fridge so that it's there when you finally stop for lunch.

Stock up on some of the great instant soups, stews, and curries available at your natural foods store. These cup-of-soup style products are often surprisingly tasty, and all you need is hot water from the water cooler in your office or dorm. Just don't make a steady diet of them; they're usually loaded with sodium.

Have dessert with your lunch! Enjoy leftover bread or rice pudding from last night's dinner, or a couple of vegan chocolate chip cookies. Always include a piece of fresh fruit for a sweet treat.

Any combination of foods you like as snacks can add up to a great lunch. Try two or three—or more—of the following:

- Hummus and carrot sticks
- Veggie and soy-free cheese wraps
- Trail mix
- Yogurt and fruit/granola
- Granola bars
- Muffins
- Leftover spaghetti or lasagna
- Veggie hot dogs
- Bean burritos
- Whole wheat bagels
- Vegetarian sloppy joes
- Pasta salad
- Sushi
- Cereal and hemp milk
- Potato salad or coleslaw
- Popcorn with nutritional yeast seasoning
- Black olives
- Leftover Chinese food
- Bean dip with tortilla chips

Planning Your Meals—Dinner

Dinnertime is one of the most squandered parts of our day. We're tired, we've been busy, we may not have a lot of time, so we grab something and eat it in front of the TV or computer. If you have roommates or live with your family, try making mealtime a ritual of togetherness. Work together to prepare it, sit down and savor it, and use this time to catch up on your day,

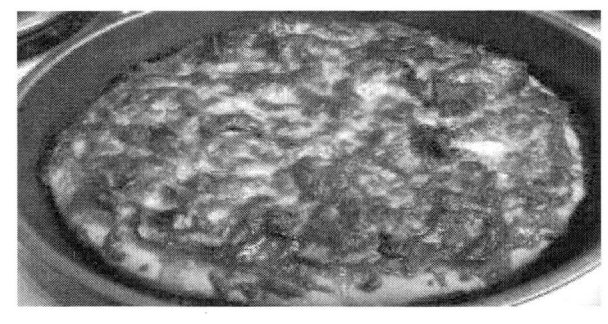

Use dinnertime to experiment with new twists on old favorites. Substitute portabella mushrooms and sautéed onions for the ground beef in your favorite lasagna, or make a great vegetarian chili.

Make a big pot of soup on the weekend and refrigerate or freeze portions of easy weekday meals. By cooking more elaborate dishes when you're relaxed and have the time, you can prepare for a hectic week by stocking up on homemade, heat-and-eat dinners.

Once a week, make a list of the dinners you'd like to have during the week and buy all the ingredients during a trip to the store. Be realistic. On nights that you know you'll be working late or feeling extra tired, choose meals that are easy to prepare. Then post the list on your refrigerator, so you're committed to making that meal! This will keep you from grabbing a peanut butter sandwich just because you don't know what to eat!

Planning Your Meals: Snacks

Snacking is a part of life. Everyone snacks, whether between meals or in the evening. Sticking to your vegetarian diet when it comes to snacking is a lot easier than people think. Having a midmorning or an afternoon snack is a good way to avoid hunger pangs later on, which might cause you to overeat at lunch or dinner. Snacks also help you maintain a healthy metabolism as well as a healthy eating schedule. And as a vegetarian, you have a wide variety of snacks to choose from.

Some sensible vegetarian snack ideas include:

> Rice milk and fruit smoothie
> Cookies and rice milk
> Graham crackers and rice milk
> Fruit
> Fruit salad
> Oatmeal cookies
> Fig Newtons
> Rice pudding
> Frozen fruit bars
> Yogurt
> Bran muffin
> English muffin
> Wheat toast and peanut butter
> Cereal with rice milk
> Bagel with jelly

If you simply take the time to glance around your cupboards and refrigerator, you'll easily find many more snack ideas to add to the list.

Planning ahead can help you keep on track with your meal plans and schedule. It will also keep you from excuses such as "there's not enough time to cook a meal" or, "I don't have the right foods to make dinner." Excuses like these can easily lead to slipups and poor meal choices. One rule of thumb for planning ahead when it comes to a vegetarian diet is to prepare food that can be stored in the refrigerator or freezer and eaten at a later date. Set aside a few hours on the weekend to prepare three or four meals for the upcoming week. Having ready-made meals available to eat is key, because when you are too tired or too busy to cook, you'll be able to stick to your vegetarian diet.

Here is a list of foods that can be made and then stored in the refrigerator to serve as ready-made meals:

> Coleslaw
> Cucumber and tomato salad

Fruit salad
Hummus
Potato salad
Three bean salad
Black bean salad
Black bean dip
Fresh salsa
Vegetable salad with leafy greens

Here is a list of foods that can be made and then stored in the freezer to serve as ready-made meals:

Soups
Vegetable lasagna
Pesto (for pasta)
Any type of vegetable casserole
Fruit salad
Vegetarian chili
Moroccan chili
Lentil chili

You can also freeze breads, muffins, cookies, and other bread products. Keep them in small plastic bags that you can easily grab if you are in a hurry or on the go!

CHAPTER 13

Delicious Vegetarian Recipes that Everyone Can Enjoy

There are tons of great recipe books for vegetarians, including veggie123.com cookbook[1]. It's not difficult to find recipes, and you can always adapt your favorites to your new lifestyle. You can almost always find a viable substitute for any meat product in a recipe. This is where experimentation comes into play. You can have fun by trying out different substitutes to see which ones works and tastes the best. For example, instead of using eggs when making a cake, you can use applesauce, rice milk, or fruit juice instead.

Whenever you come across a recipe that calls for meat products, play around with it. Take down notes on the vegetarian substitutes you decide to use and which ones work the best. Then you can use that recipe again whenever you like except this time it will have a fun, new vegetarian twist.

Before you start experimenting though, here are some vegetarian recipes to get you started. All of them are good for ovo-lacto-vegetarians. The vegan recipes are noted as such, and ovo-lactos can enjoy them too!

Breakfast

Old-Style Potato Pancakes
Serves 8

        4 medium baking potatoes, peeled and coarsely shredded

---

1 medium onion, coarsely shredded
4 green onions, chopped
1 egg, beaten
salt and pepper to taste
vegetable oil for frying

In a large bowl, mix the potatoes and onions. Wrap the mixture in cheesecloth or paper towels, and squeeze out the excess liquid into another bowl. The starch from the potatoes will settle into the bottom of the bowl. Pour out the water, and save the remaining potato starch.

In a large bowl, combine the potato mixture, green onions, egg, salt and pepper, and reserved potato starch. Coat a nonstick 12-inch skillet or griddle with a in layer of oil and heat it over medium-high heat. For each pancake, press together about 2 tablespoons of the potato mixture with your hands, place it on the skillet, and flatten it with a heat-proof spatula. Cook for about 8 minutes, turning once, until brown on both sides. Serve hot.

Savory Breakfast Flan
Serves 6

Ingredients:

6 oz. grated cheddar cheese, plus two tablespoons
8 oz. frozen corn
10 eggs
1 teaspoon salt
1 teaspoon pepper
1/4 teaspoon nutmeg
Dash cayenne
1 1/4 cup skim milk
3/4 cup half-and-half

Spray a 9"x13" baking pan with cooking spray. Spread half of the cheese in the bottom of the pan. Layer half of the corn on top of the cheese layer. Repeat with layers of cheese and corn. Combine all remaining ingredients except the 2 tablespoons cheddar, and pour over corn and cheese. Bake at 325°F for 1 hour, or until puffy and lightly browned. Sprinkle with remaining 2 tablespoons shredded cheddar and return to oven for 1 minute. Run a sharp knife around edges to loosen, cut into rectangles, and serve.

Oatmeal Spice Breakfast Bars (vegan)
Makes about 10 bars

> 2 2/3 cups rolled oats
> 1/3 cup flaxseed meal
> 2 medium bananas, mashed
> 1/3 cup canola oil
> 1 cup dried fruit, in any combination (raisins, dates, cherries, and cranberries are good)
> 2/3 cup chopped nuts or sunflower seeds
> 1 tsp. cinnamon
> 1/4 tsp. nutmeg
> 1/4 tsp. ginger
> 2 Tbsp. sweetener, or more to taste (nonvegans may use honey)
> Vegan egg substitute product to equal one egg

Combine all the dry ingredients and mix well. Add bananas, egg substitute, oil, and sweetener; combine until blended and mixture is sticky. If the mixture appears to dry, add a small amount of water. Shape dough into 1/2-inch thick bars on a greased cookie sheet. Bake at 350°F for 15 minutes.

Easy Vegan Pancakes
Serves 4 to 6

> 2 cups whole-wheat flour
> 1 tsp. baking soda
> 1 tsp. baking powder
> 2 cups vanilla rice milk
> 1 tsp. cinnamon
> 2 Tbsp. vegetable oil

Combine flour, baking soda, and baking powder. Add milk and oil, stirring until just mixed (it should still be a little lumpy). Heat skillet until a drop of cold water dances across the surface; grease pan with spray oil and drop 1/4 to 1 cup batter onto skillet for each pancake.

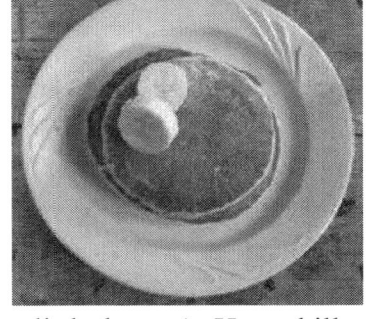

When the edges look brown and the air bubbles appear on the top of the pancake, turn and cook the other side. Serve with syrup or fresh fruit.

Carrot Breakfast Muffins (vegan)
Serves 6 to 8

    1 cup whole-wheat flour
    1 cup oat bran
    1 Tbsp. cornstarch
    1 tsp. baking soda
    1 tsp. baking powder
    1 tsp. cinnamon
    1 tsp. nutmeg
    1/3 tsp. ginger
    2/3 cup grated carrots
    1/3 cup maple syrup
    1 cup water
    1/4 cup canola oil

Preheat the oven to 375°F. In a large mixing bowl, combine all of the dry ingredients and the grated carrots. Add all of the wet ingredients. Mix well. Pour the batter into a lightly oiled muffin pan, and bake for 25 to 30 minutes, or until an inserted toothpick comes out clean.

Other breakfast options:

Breakfast Burritos: Eggs or chickpeas scrambled with onions, peppers and chopped vegetarian sausage, topped with cheese and rolled up in a warm tortilla.

McVegetarian Sandwich: Place scrambled eggs (or egg substitute, or chickpeas), vegetarian faux-Canadian bacon, and cheese in a sliced English muffin. A great take-and-eat breakfast!

Cereal Free-For-All: Mix two, three, or more of your favorite cold cereals in a bowl for a different twist on your usual breakfast.

Lunch

Quinoa Salad

Serves 4 to 6

    1 1/2 cups quinoa
    3 cups water
    2 bell peppers (green or red, or combination), diced
    1 cup diced red onion
    1 cup finely chopped fresh dill
    1/4 cup balsamic vinegar
    2 tablespoons sweetener, or to taste (non-vegans may use honey)
    1 tablespoon Dijon mustard

Rinse the quinoa well to remove outer coating. Add quinoa and water to medium saucepan. Bring to a boil, cover, and simmer over low heat for 15 minutes, or until all the liquid has been absorbed. Combine peppers, onion, and dill in a medium mixing bowl. Add cooked quinoa. In a separate bowl, combine remaining ingredients. Add to quinoa mixture and toss gently. Add salt and pepper to taste. Cover and chill for 2 hours before serving.

Cheese-Free Mac 'n Cheese (vegan)
Serves 4 to 6

    1 package (16 oz) elbow macaroni
    2 cups vanilla rice milk
    2 tablespoons soy-free margarine
    2 tablespoons vegan mayonnaise
    1 cup nutritional yeast
    1 tsp. salt
    1 tsp. white pepper
    1 tsp. garlic powder
    1 tsp. hot sauce (optional)
    1 tsp. turmeric optional(adds yellow color)

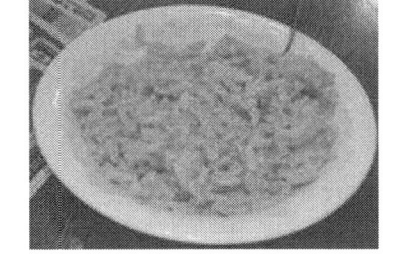

Cook pasta according to package directions; drain. In a large bowl, combine pasta with other ingredients. Mix thoroughly.

Optional: For more flavor and an added nutritional boost, add 1 cup of steamed broccoli.

Sloppy Faux-Joes (vegan)
Serves 4 to 6

>1 large onion, diced
>2 medium green peppers, diced
>3 Tbsp. olive oil
>1 cup boiling water
>2 cups tomato purée
>Freshly ground pepper, to taste
>1 Tbsp. soy sauce
>1 Tbsp. mustard
>1 Tbsp. sugar
>1 cup dry textured vegetable protein (TVP)
>2 tsp. chili powder
>vegan buns

In a large skillet, sauté onion and green peppers in the olive oil until soft, about 12 minutes. Add the remaining ingredients (except buns), and simmer over low heat for 20 minutes, stirring often. Serve in buns for sandwiches, or spoon over bread for less sloppy eating with a fork.

Hummus Garden Pita
Serves 1 or 2

>1 medium firm ripe tomato, finely diced
>1/4 cup seeded cucumber or bell pepper, diced
>1 cup shredded lettuce
>Creamy vegetarian salad dressing (your favorite)
>1/4 cup hummus
>1 regular-size or 2 mini pita breads, cut in half

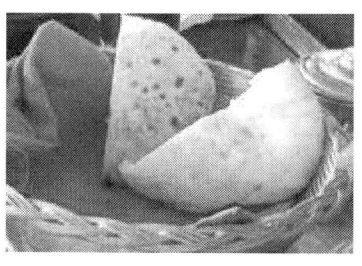

Combine the tomato, cucumber, or pepper and lettuce in a medium bowl. Add enough dressing to moisten and toss. Spread the inside of the pita with hummus, then fill with salad. To take with you to school or work, wrap first in foil, then in plastic zipper bags.

Dinner

Black Bean Burritos (vegan)
Serves 4

> 1 15-ounce can black beans, drained and rinsed well
> 1/4 cup salsa
> 1 cup cooked brown rice
> 4 flour tortillas (vegetarian style, of course)
> 1 cup shredded leaf or spinach
> 1 tomato, diced
> 1 avocado, diced or mashed

Combine the black beans, salsa, and rice in a saucepan, and simmer for 3 minutes, stirring occasionally. Remove from heat, cover, and let sit for 5 minutes. In an ungreased skillet, heat a tortilla until warm. Spread a line of the bean mixture down the center. Top with lettuce, tomato, avocado, and more salsa, if desired. Roll up.

Optional: Nonvegans may add sour cream.

Vegetarian Moussaka
Serves 8 to 10

> 1 eggplant, thinly sliced
> 1 Tbsp. olive oil
> 1 large zucchini, thinly sliced
> 2 potatoes, thinly sliced
> 1 onion, sliced
> 1 clove garlic, chopped
> 1 Tbsp. white vinegar
> 1 (14.5 ounce) can whole peeled tomatoes, chopped
> 1 (14.5 ounce) can lentils, drained, juice reserved
> 1 teaspoon dried oregano
> 2 Tbsp. chopped fresh parsley
> Salt and pepper to taste
> 1 cup crumbled feta cheese
> 1 Tbsp. butter
> 2 Tbsp. all-purpose flour
> 1 1/4 cups milk
> black pepper to taste
> 1 pinch ground nutmeg

1 egg, beaten
1/4 cup grated Parmesan cheese

Sprinkle eggplant slices with salt, and set aside for 30 minutes. Rinse and pat dry. Preheat oven to 375°F. Heat oil in a large skillet over medium-high heat. Lightly brown eggplant and zucchini slices on both sides; drain. Adding more oil if necessary, brown potato slices; drain. Sauté onion and garlic until lightly browned. Pour in vinegar and reduce heat. Stir in tomatoes, lentils, half of the juice from lentils, oregano, and parsley. Cover; reduce heat to medium-low, and simmer for 15 minutes.

In a 9×13-inch casserole, dish layer eggplant, zucchini, potatoes, onions, and feta. Pour tomato mixture over vegetables; repeat layering, finishing with a layer of eggplant and zucchini. Cover and bake in preheated oven for 25 minutes. Meanwhile, in a small saucepan, combine butter, flour, and milk. Bring to a slow boil, whisking constantly until thick and smooth. Season with pepper and add nutmeg. Remove from heat, cool for 5 minutes, and stir in beaten egg. Pour sauce over vegetables and sprinkle with Parmesan cheese. Bake, uncovered, for another 25 to 30 minutes.

Easy Vegetarian Chili (vegan)
Serves 6

1 small onion, chopped
1 large green bell pepper, seeded and chopped
3/4 cup chopped celery
3/4 cup dry red wine or water
3 cloves garlic, finely chopped
2 (14.5-ounce) cans diced tomatoes, undrained
1 cup water
1/4 cup tomato paste
3 tsp. vegetable bouillon granules
1 Tbsp. chili powder
1 tsp. ground cumin
1 tsp. cinnamon
2 tsp. paprika

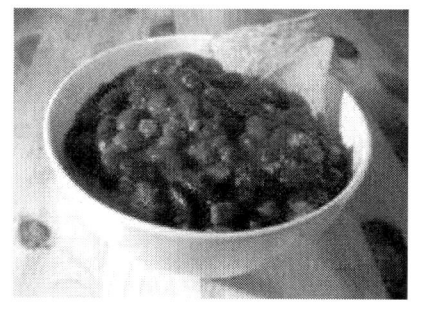

1 tsp. cayenne (red) pepper
2 (15-ounce) cans kidney or pinto beans, rinsed and drained
Sour cream (optional)

Combine onion, bell pepper, celery, wine, and garlic in large saucepan. Cook over medium-high heat, stirring occasionally, for 6 to 8 minutes or until vegetables are tender. Add tomatoes with juice, water, tomato paste, and bouillon; bring to a boil. Reduce heat to simmer and add chili powder, cumin, cinnamon, paprika, and cayenne. Stir in beans. Reduce heat to low; simmer, stirring occasionally, for 45 minutes. Add beans during the last 15 minutes of cooking. Nonvegans may serve with sour cream.

Other great dinner ideas:

Vegetarian Lasagna: Adapt your favorite homemade lasagna recipe by adding a package of frozen chopped spinach (well-drained with moisture squeezed out) to the ricotta layer. Use vegetarian marinara sauce.

Layered Crock Pot Dinner: Layer veggies in the crock pot in this order—sliced potatoes on the bottom, then sliced onions, sliced carrots, sliced bell pepper, sliced zucchini, and 1 cup each of corn and peas. Gently pour over this a sauce made from 2 cups tomato sauce, 1/4 cup low-sodium tamari soy sauce, and 1 teaspoon each of thyme, dry mustard, basil, chili powder, cinnamon, sage, and parsley. Cook for six hours on low or 12 hours on high. A great meal to come home to at the end of a busy day!

Artichoke Pate: Toss a jar of marinated artichoke hearts into the food processor with a cup of walnuts, a clove of garlic, 3 ounces olive oil, 2 tablespoons of lemon juice, and a teaspoon each of salt, pepper, rosemary and basil. Process until smooth, and serve on cracker or whole wheat bread.

CHAPTER 14

Shopping in the Health Food Aisle

Solving the Mysteries of Seeds, Soy, and Stevia

We've talked a little bit about meat substitutes, including grains like quinoa ... but what are they? What do you use them for? And where the heck do you get them? Luckily, as more and more people become vegetarian (and nonvegetarians cut back on animal foods), more co-ops and whole foods stores keep cropping up, even in smaller towns. Mainstream grocery stores keep expanding their natural foods sections because customers are demanding whole-grain products. It's just a matter of knowing what you're buying and what are all the delicious ways you can add variety to your vegetarian diet.

Tofu for You

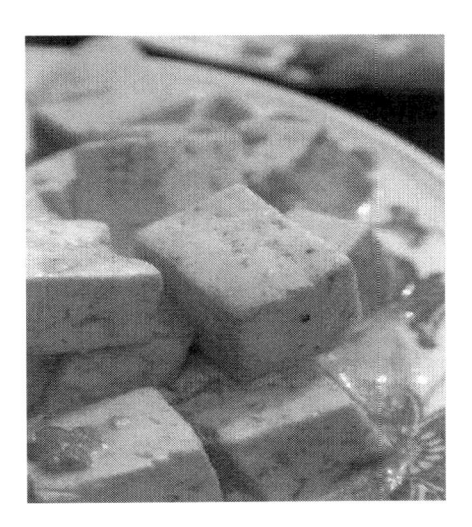

The two most common meat-substitute protein foods you'll find in vegetarian cooking are tofu and tempeh, but they're very different from each other. As we begin to discuss tofu, it's important to note that there are a lot of health concerns that surround this unique food. One of the most important is the potential thyroid problems that can be caused by too much soy. Some people experience this right off the bat, and some experience it after a number of years. However, once experienced, it's far too late to rectify the situation.

While some vegetarian diets revolve wholly around tofu, the potential health concerns probably outweigh the benefits of this food, so it's best to avoid it if possible. Understanding its role in the diets of others, though, may help you as you get started.

Tofu is a smooth, almost flavorless curd made from soybeans. While Westerners still think of tofu as exotic or as a strictly vegetarian food, it's been a staple in other countries' cuisine for thousands of years. The Chinese have been eating tofu since at least 200 BC, and it's used every day in Asian homes. Bean curd is another term for tofu, so keep an eye out in Chinese restaurants for menu items that feature curd—it may be tofu!

Tofu is made from soymilk in a manner similar to the way cheese is manufactured from animal milk. A curdling agent is added to the soy, causing the solid matter to clump into curds. The curds are then pressed into a solid block.

The flavor-free quality of tofu is precisely what makes it so versatile. Tofu is spongy and porous, and absorbs other flavors very well, so it can be adapted to almost any kind of dish. It comes in a variety of textures, from extra-firm to soft, so it can be used as a meat substitute and egg substitute, or it can stand in for dairy in fillings, sauces, dips, and puddings. Recipes will tell you which type to use, and once you get used to cooking with it, you'll come up with countless ideas on your own.

For a meat substitute, firm or extra-firm tofu is usually cut into cubes and added to stir-fry dishes, or marinated in soy sauce (or other flavorful liquid) and cooked in big chunks. If you freeze tofu and then defrost it, the texture becomes more chewy—a quality ideal for people who miss the texture of meat.

Silken tofu, combined with melted chocolate (vegan or otherwise) makes an excellent chocolate pudding or cream pie filling. Soft tofu can be used to make creamy sauces; just puree cooked vegetable in a blender or food processor and add tofu. This same method works to make creamy, dairy-free soups.

Whatever form it takes, it was once considered a marvelous source of nutrition. Primarily eaten as a high-quality source of protein, tofu that's been processed with calcium salt is also a source of calcium. It also contains iron and other minerals. It is fairly high in fat, but it is actually free of cholesterol and generally lower in fat than animal proteins. There are also lower fat tofu products on the market. Firm tofu is usually higher in fat than soft tofu.

Because of its soft consistency and bland taste, tofu was once considered a good source of nutrition for babies or older people who had difficulty chewing hard foods. It's most commonly sold in tubs or vacuum packs and can be found in either the dairy case or produce section of your supermarket. Once opened, leftover tofu may be stored by rinsing, covering with fresh water daily, and placed in the refrigerator, where it will keep for up to a week. Tofu can be frozen for up to five months.

Giving in to Tem(peh)tation

Tempeh is a more strongly flavored soy product made from fermented soybeans and sometimes containing other grains like rice or millet. Like tofu, it's another ancient food, with uses dating back to Indonesia some two thousand years ago. It's not as creamy or as versatile as tofu, and comes in patties; it's recognizable by its pale brown, rough texture.

But don't let tempeh's forbidding appearance stop you from trying it. It's great as a substitute for meat on dishes that traditionally call for animal proteins. It has a delicious nutty flavor, and you can crumble it into pita sandwiches or chili, or make "chicken salad" with tempeh in place of poultry. If you're feeling creative, it can also be grilled, baked, barbecued, or skewered with veggies for a tempeh kabob. It's also great in soups, stews, or casseroles.

Tempeh is generally available in shrink-wrap packages or reusable plastic bags. Like tofu, it's high in protein and fat, but is also cholesterol-free.

What's the Truth about Soy?

For a little while, soy products were at the top of the vegetarian hierarchy and were often celebrated as the perfect meat substitute. (Tempeh is safer to consume because of the fermentation process.) In the past decade, they have enjoyed favorable press. So what happened? Why are soy products suddenly being vilified and labeled dangerous? Well, many antisoy advocates claimed that eating soy raised the risk of cancer, osteoporosis, thyroid problems, birth defects, reproductive problems, nutritional deficiencies, and Alzheimer's disease. The consumer was left to ponder who was right—the soy proponents or the soy bashers?

First, it's significant to note that the soybean has been around for ages and was often used for food for thousands of years. But with the vegetarian movement in full swing, especially in North America, soy has been implemented in meat substitutes, protein beverages, chips, ice cream, yogurt, and other products. It's plain to see that soy is everywhere, so the consideration of the safety of soy is an important one. Here are the most common concerns:

Soy increases the risk of cancer. One of the first endorsements of soy was the fact that it reduced the incidence of cancer. Now, antisoy advocates are saying the opposite. Studies have been mixed, but some have shown that soy products can in fact raise the risk of cancer. It's always better to be mindful of the risks involved in any situation, especially serious health risks.

Soy will interfere with thyroid function. It is true that soy contains goitrogens, as do many other foods such as cruciferous vegetables (cabbage, cauliflower, broccoli, and brussel sprouts), sweet potatoes, lima beans, and millet. However, soy does not cause thyroid problems in healthy, well-nourished people who are not deficient in iodine. Still, knowing that soy products do contain goitrogens should be enough to be cautious.

Soyfoods will cause mental problems and age-related issues. Evidence suggests that soy offers some benefits to mental stability and function, though its effect on older individuals is still under investigation. There have been studies done on mental deterioration when too much soy is consumed.

If you are determined to eat soy regardless of the information provided above, that is your choice. Just remember that moderation is the key. It is my recommendation that you avoid soy products altogether. There are other alternatives.

Soy alternatives include:

Wheat grains—This is your best nonsoy alternative because they are high in protein.

Pastas—Choose nonbleached pasta for the most healthful option. Add protein-rich vegetables to your pasta for additional benefits and better flavor.

Cereals—Certain cereals are rich in protein and offer a great way to get a good start on the day. Since you can't drink soymilk with them, consider rice milk or another milk alternative.

Protein-rich vegetables—The vegetables you'll want to stock up on for protein purposes include leeks, parsley, chives, and red and green peppers.

Seaweed—Seaweed deserves a category of its own because it is such a popular nonsoy choice for proteins. It is added to vegan shakes to boost proteins or can be consumed on its own.

Nuts—Nuts are another good choice to add to your daily diet to get the protein you need.

Seeds—Seeds can be eaten alone as snacks, combined into trail mix, added as a topping to salads, and used as an ingredient in entrees.

As you can see, there are plenty of alternatives to soy. You don't have to risk increasing your chances of getting cancer, mental deterioration, or thyroid problems in order to stick to you vegetarian diet. All you have to do is be aware of what you are eating. The rest is cake!

Seize the Seitan

Seitan is a brown, chewy protein food (pronounced SAY-tahn) that's made from gluten, the protein portion of wheat. If you live in a small town, it may be difficult to find. It's usually only available in natural food stores. It can be purchased as a mix, but it's most commonly purchased ready-made.

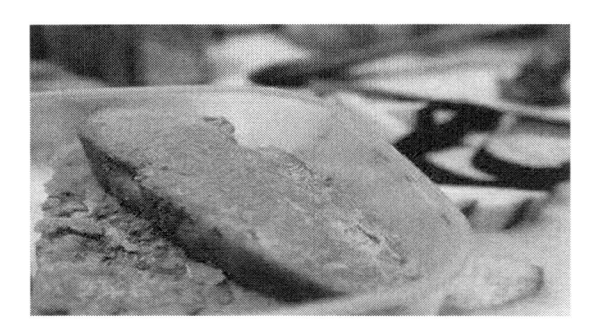

If you've never had seitan, try it the next time you're at a Thai or Chinese restaurant, served in a stir-fry or other dish. It's delicious and a terrific low-fat source of protein. Once you try it, you'll want to use it in sandwiches, simmered in vegetable broth or baked in the oven; the texture is different depending on how it's prepared. It's also excellent as a substitute for beef in Stroganoff.

Those Great Grains

As you stroll the aisles of your natural foods store, you'll find a treasure trove of grains with exotic names and a wide variety of textures that you never ever knew existed. Whole grains are a vital part of the vegetarian diet, and learning how to use different grains in your cooking will add variety and excitement to your menus.

Just the different types of rice take up several shelves at a good health food store. You'll find short, medium, and long-grain white and brown rice, arborio rice, sushi rice, jasmine rice, sweet rice, and white and brown basmati rice. Then there are the whole grains—amaranth, barley, buckwheat, bulgur, cornmeal, *kamut*, millet, oats, quinoa, spelt, and more. All have different tastes and textures, and all deserve a chance to shine on your dinner table.

Before cooking whole grains, rinse them thoroughly to remove dirt and debris, especially if you are buying from bulk bins (and you should buy in bulk whenever you can—it costs less). Some grains, like quinoa, need to be rinsed to remove their bitter outer coating. To cook them, use a heavy nonaluminum pot (some grains interact with the aluminum) with a tight-fitting lid. Cover the grains with cold water, and stir gently to separate the grains. Bring the water to a boil—with a pinch of salt, if you like—then lower the heat to a simmer and cook, covered, until done.

Cooking times (by grain):

GRAIN (1 cup dry)	WATER (salted) (cups)	COOKING TIME (minutes)	YIELD (cups)
Amaranth	2	25–30	2–2
Barley, whole/hulled	3	90	3–4
Barley, pearled	3	45	3–4
Buckwheat groats	2	15	2–2
Corn grits	3	20	3–4
Kamut	3	120	2–3/4
Millet	2	25	3–4
Oats, whole	3	60	3
Oats, rolled (oatmeal)	2	15	1–2

Quinoa	2	20	3–3
RICE:			
Arborio	2	30	2–2
Basmati, brown	2	45	3
Brown	2	45	2–3
Sushi	2	45	2
Sweet	1	45	2
Spelt	3	90–120	2
WHEAT:			
Whole berries	3	90–120	2
Bulgur	2	15	2
Couscous	2	1	2–3

Grains are delicious, nutritious, and versatile foods, and great sources of fiber. Because of this, they're very chewy, so make sure you eat slowly, thoughtfully, and thoroughly for proper digestion. Grains rushed through the system can cause gas and bloating, so slow down and enjoy your food!

Nuts about Nuts—and Seeds

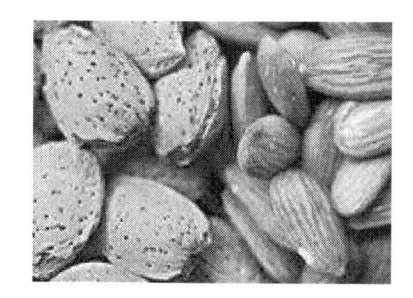

Almonds come on two varieties, the bitter almond and the sweet almond. Both are native to the Middle East, but are also grown widely in Europe and the Americas. The Romans considered almonds a sign of fertility and prosperity, and gave them as wedding gifts—remember that the next time you get that little bag of Jordan almonds at a reception! In cooking, bitter almonds are used to manufacture almond oil, while sweet almonds are used for cooking and eating raw. They're very nutritious, loaded with magnesium, phosphorous, zinc, calcium, folic acid, and vitamin E.

The **Brazil nut** is the big one in your grandmother's nut bowl, the one that's a challenge to crack open. They're actually the seeds of a tree that grows up to five-feet tall in the Amazon jungle, and they're harvested from seedpod clusters that look a little like coconuts. Commercially, Brazil nuts are still harvested from wild trees, so keep that in mind when you buy them. Some environmentalists believe they're being overharvested. Shelled Brazil nuts are tasty snacks, and they can be used in dessert recipes too.

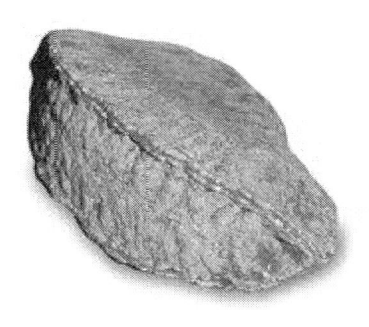

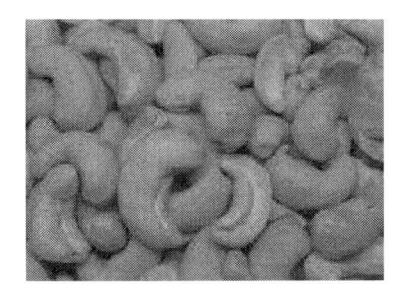

Cashews grow beneath a fleshy plant called the "cashew pear" whose fruit can be used to make juices, syrups and liqueurs. Eaten alone or in savory dishes or candy, they're a great source of vitamin A.

Hazelnuts grow in Europe and the UnitedStates, although most of the world's hazelnuts come from Turkey. Round or oval with a very hard shell, they grow in clusters and are partially enclosed in a husk. Hazelnuts are a very nutritious snack, as they're high in fiber, potassium, calcium, magnesium, and vitamin E. Used in candies, baked foods, and savory dishes, they can be a bit of a chore to cook with. The raw hazelnuts must be roasted in the oven first to loosen their papery skin, then rubbed inside a clean kitchen towel to remove the entire coating.

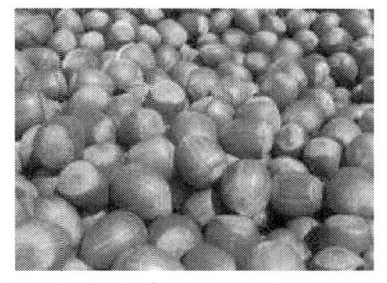

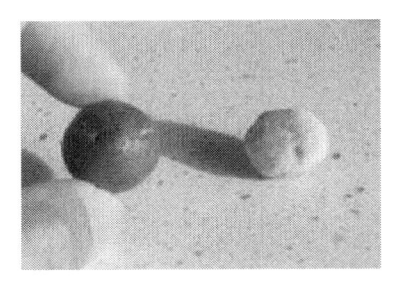

Macadamias originate in Australia but are now grown commercially in Hawaii for the American market. It's widely used in cookies, candies, and ice cream, and is sold as a salty snack food. Commercial cultivation of macadamias began in 1858. It is named after John McAdam, who first cultivated it. Low in carbohydrates but quite high in fat, they're a good source of calcium and other minerals.

Peanuts really are members of the pea family and aren't actually nuts at all, as they grow in the ground instead on trees. Also known as "groundnuts," peanuts are very nutritious, with a high protein and oil content plus lots of vitamins B and E.

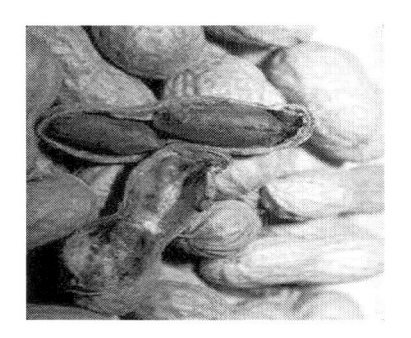

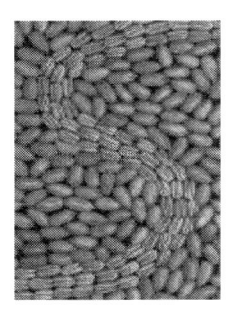

Pecans are native to North America, and were an important food source for the native Indian tribes. They belong to the same family as the walnut, but are slightly sweeter. And they're good for you, rich in vitamins A, B, and E, calcium, phosphorous, magnesium, potassium, and zinc. Use them in cookies, cakes, and other baked foods, eat them alone, or chop them up and add them to hot cereal.

Pine nuts (also called pignolas) are the seeds of the stone pine tree and are widely used in Mediterranean cuisine. As a source of protein, the pine nuts are used in many different dishes, most notably pesto sauce—a processed combination of fresh basil leaves, olive oil, and pine nuts.

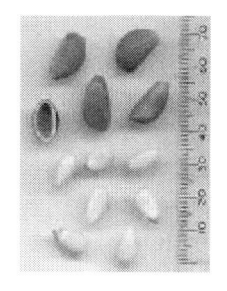

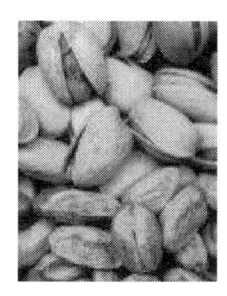

Pistachios were first cultivated over a hundred thousand years ago in Iran and Syria, and then brought to Europe. Because of its open shell, pistachios are easily roasted and salted, and are usually eaten as peel-and-eat snacks. Pistachios were originally dyed red by importers to hide imperfections on their shells that occurred when they were picked by hand. The scare over Red Dye #2 in the 1970s put a stop to that practice for a while, allowing customers to realize that pistachios aren't naturally red in color. They're harvested by machine now, so the dye is unnecessary. But some companies use a harmless red color on pistachios' shells because customers expect them to be red! Pistachios are rich in calcium, magnesium, phosphorous, potassium, iron, folic acid, and protein.

Walnuts come in over fifteen different varieties, but the most popular is the English walnut. Walnuts originated in southeast Europe and central Asia, and are now grown commercially throughout Europe and the Americas. Historians believe that there was a walnut grove in the famed Hanging Gardens of Babylon. Because of the walnut's resemblance to a human brain, it was once believed to cure headaches. And maybe they helped, as they're a great source of phosphorous, potassium, and magnesium as well as proteins and vitamin E. Walnuts are a classic addition to countless sweet and savory recipes, and can be eaten raw; they can even be pickled when harvested while still green.

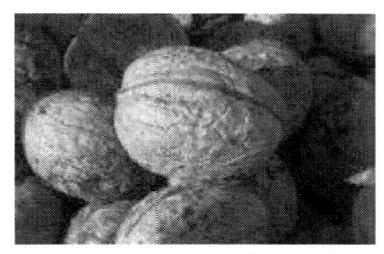

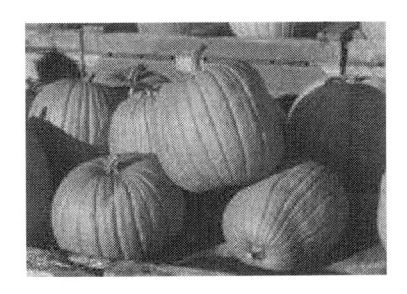

Pumpkin seeds can be eaten raw or used in a variety of sweet and savory recipes. They're rich in protein, iron, zinc, and phosphorous. During the fall when they're in season, you can dry your own pumpkin seeds. They're delicious roasted and sprinkled with salt or soy sauce while hot, served on salads, or added to baked foods.

Sesame seeds originated in Africa but are now commonly grown in many tropical and subtropical areas. Oil is extracted from the seed and used for cooking, and as an addition to salad oil, commercial margarines, and salad dressings. Toasted sesame oil, available in Chinese markets and the ethnic aisle of your supermarket, is a tasty addition to veggie stir-fries and rice dishes. The seeds are used in cakes, cookies, and candies (as well as the ubiquitous sesame seed hamburger buns) and are often sprinkled as a garnish on oriental foods. Sesame seed paste (tahini) is a must-have food for the vegetarian, and it's an ingredient in hummus. The delicious sweet treat halvah is made from sesame seeds. Sesame seeds are also a particularly good source of protein and calcium.

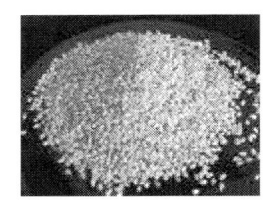

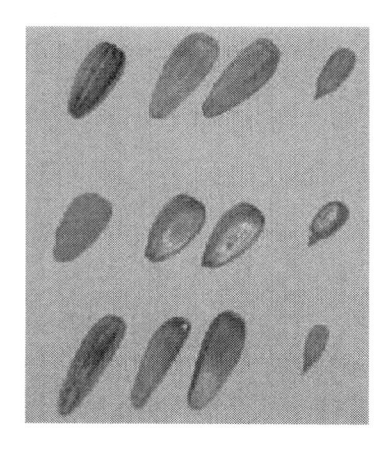

Sunflower seeds are widely available, and a popular snack item. The sunflower is a member of the daisy family, and originated in North America or Mexico, where Native Americans cultivated them over two thousand years ago. They're a fine source of potassium and phosphorous, and contain protein, iron, and calcium. The seeds can be eaten whole, raw, or cooked, and they're a crunchy addition to breads and cakes, or sprinkled over salads or breakfast cereals.

Low-calorie Sweetness the Natural Way

Chances are you've never heard of stevia or, if you have, you know little about it. For people dedicated to eating well, it's a valuable tool, but there are powerful people who would rather you were kept in the dark.

Every year in the United States, over five thousand food products are sold which are artificially sweetened. If you're diabetic, hypoglycemic, or trying to lose weight, you probably buy these products. The sweeteners most commonly used are saccharin, acesulfame-K, and aspartame. These chemical sweeteners are in everything from chewing gum and soft drinks to children's multivitamins. Designed in laboratories, made in giant chemical factories, and sold by multibillion-dollar conglomerates, they go by innocent-sounding names like NutraSweet, Sweet n' Low, and Equal, and they carry almost no warnings about their possible dangers.

If you look closely at packages of aspartame, you'll see no warning that the substance has caused brain tumors in laboratory animals. And the National Cancer Institute has seen an increase in the incidence of malignant brain tumors in Americans since the introduction of aspartame in the early 1980s. Many people complain about headaches after eating foods sweetened with aspartame. Coincidence? In fact, thousands of people have registered over ninety-two different side effects related to aspartame with the FDA and the Centers for Disease Control, including headaches, menstrual irregularities, nausea, dizziness, skin lesions, rashes, hyperactivity, heart palpitations, gastrointestinal disorders, blackouts, numbness, memory loss, blindness, seizures, and suicidal depression. And those are just the ones that have been reported—a small percentage of the number of people who experience these symptoms.

There's a lengthy history behind the FDA's approval of aspartame, but the condensed version is this: despite there being a lot of tests that showed that aspartame was potentially dangerous, it was approved for sale. In 1985, Ohio Senator Howard Metzenbaum tried to pass a bill requiring studies into the safety of aspartame, but the Labor and Human Resources Committee stopped it instead. And despite there being strong evidence to suggest that aspartame works like a neurotoxin, actually changing brain chemistry and interacting with other drugs, there's no regulation on it. It's present in thousands of products consumed by mean, women, children, and the elderly every day.

Stevia Rebaudiana Bertoni is a perennial shrub native to Paraguay, and it's been used as a natural sweetener by the Guarani Indians for hundreds of years; they use it primarily to sweeten their herbal *mat* tea. South American settlers in Paraguay, Argentina, and Brazil began using it in the 1800s, and around 1908, plantations started cultivating stevia for commercial purposes. Over the next several decades, botanists and businessmen attempted to interest the U.S. government in cultivating stevia for the domestic market, but sugar producers managed to keep them from making any headway.

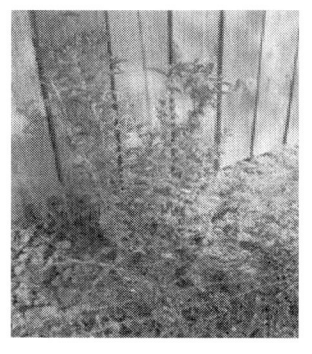

In the 1970s the Japanese, who had already banned aspartame, discovered stevia, and some American companies used it in their herbal teas in the 1980s. It looked like stevia was finally poised to reach the American consumer—except that the FDA began taking action against companies that were using stevia, including embargoes, search and seizures, and calling for an import alert on the sweetener. Stevia was denied the all-important FDA "generally recognized as safe" status, despite it's long history of scientific studies supporting its safety. At about the same time that the FDA was granting the corporate giant G.D. Searle's request to allow aspartame to be used in dry foods and beverages, stevia—a completely natural and safe substance with no side effects whatsoever—was classified as an "unsafe food additive," and Celestial Seasonings and other companies were forced to stop using stevia.

Despite the FDA's long-held opposition to stevia—and a bizarre period in 1998 when the FDA actually demanded that a Texas importer destroy a warehouse full of stevia-recipe cookbooks—it has been allowed to enter the United States as a food supplement. This completely natural, nontoxic, noncaloric sweetener, that's enjoyed by people all over the world, is a threat to the big corporate chemical sweetener companies for several reasons:

Stevia actually balances blood sugar levels and is safe for use by both diabetics and hypoglycemics.

Unlike aspartame, there are *no reports of adverse effects* from stevia's use, and scientific studies throughout the world prove its safety.

Unlike aspartame, stevia *reduces the craving for sweets*; this makes it an ideal sweetener for people trying to lose weight.

Unlike sugar, stevia *reduces cavities* by retarding the growth of plaque.

Still not convinced? Pick some up at your health food store; it's available in powder or liquid form.

CHAPTER 15

The Pros and Cons of Milk, Cheese, Yogurt, and Other Dairy Products

We've already discussed many of the problems associated with consuming dairy, from the horrible practices of factory farming to the difficulty the body has digesting cow's milk. Well ... we're going to do it again! Because while you may choose to be an ovo-lacto-vegetarian—and that's a great step toward eating a healthy, socially responsible diet—there are still some very good reasons to limit the amount of dairy products you eat.

The Truth about Osteoporosis

You probably believe that osteoporosis, the crippling disease that results in weak, brittle bones, is caused by a deficiency of calcium. For pretty much your entire life you've heard that milk does a body good and that the only way to prevent osteoporosis is to drink lots of milk, and to eat plenty of cheese and yogurt—you know, "for healthy teeth and strong bones!"

And yet, Americans and Canadians eat more dairy products than any other country while having the highest incidence of osteoporosis. In fact throughout the world, the level of hip fractures (a symptom of osteoporosis) rises in direct relationship to how much calcium the people consume!

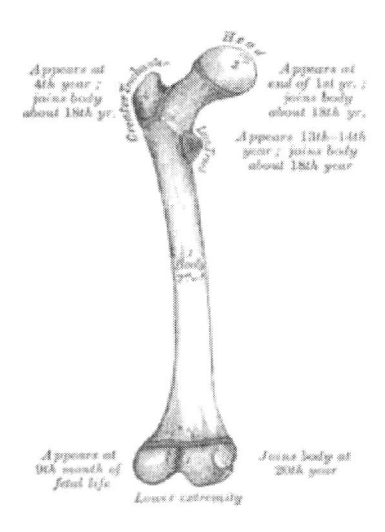

[figure: anatomical illustration of a femur bone with labels indicating ossification timing]

The truth is, like heart disease, cancer, obesity, diabetes, and a host of other ailments, osteoporosis is the by-product of affluence, not of calcium deficiency. As scientists study osteoporosis, they're discovering that it's the result of a bad, overall lifestyle, including diet. As we discussed earlier, calcium certainly plays a part in building strong bones. However, bones only build their density in our younger years, so, by the time we reach adulthood, that die has been cast. Consuming a lot of calcium as an adult simply has no bone-building effect.

Animal protein is high in sulfur-containing amino acids, which requires the body to find a way to offset the effects of those amino acids. Our bodies do this by first using the small amount of calcium in our food, then by taking it from our bones, after which point it exits the body through our urinary tract. The more meat and dairy products you eat, the more calcium you need to process them through the body. A researcher at the Creighton University School of Medicine named Robert Heaney—an advocate of dairy consumption—found in his research that the single most important factor in the rate of bone growth in young women is not how much calcium they consume, but how much calcium they consume *in relation to animal protein*. The more protein eaten, the more calcium must be consumed to offset the calcium drain. Most people in the United States, Canada, and Northern Europe eat more than twice the recommended amount of protein, and more than four or five times the amount of protein actually needed, with 70 percent of it coming from animal sources. Osteoporosis is not a result of calcium deficiency. It's a result of eating too much animal protein!

That Burning Feeling

Have you ever downed a glass of milk to sooth an upset stomach, only to find an hour later that your stomach feels bad all over again? That's because milk actually *causes* the stomach to become more acidic. Here's how it works: animal products are more difficult to digest than plant foods, which means that your stomach needs to produce more hydrochloric acid (HCI) to break them down. So let's say that you had a bowl of cereal with milk for breakfast, a little cream in your coffee, and a slice of toast with melted cheese. All that dense protein needs plenty of acid to digest it, so HCI is produced. You feel that familiar burn of acid indigestion a few hours after you eat, so you drink a glass of milk to settle your stomach. And it does, temporarily, by neutralizing the acid. But you've just added *more* animal protein to your stomach, and now your stomach will have to produce even more acid to digest it! Milk is a highly alkaline substance, so whenever you drink milk with a meal, you're actually hindering your body's ability to digest your food properly.

The Hormone Factor

If nothing else has convinced you to get your calcium from rich plant sources like broccoli, nuts, seeds, and leafy green vegetables, consider this: you're ingesting antibiotics and hormones every time you consume dairy products.

They don't call the meat and dairy industries "agribusiness" for nothing. They're businesses, and their primary goal is to make a lot of money. They make that money by selling lots and lots of animal products, and that means keeping animals healthy and growing them big. In order to do this, they pump them full of antibiotics and hormones.

Just like a nursing baby ingests whatever its mother has eaten, you consume the cow's diet when you eat animal foods. That means that you're getting hormones in your food—hormones that were used to fatten pigs and make cows give more milk, hormones to force chickens to produce more eggs and for turkeys to grow massive drumsticks.

Hormones regulate every aspect of the human body—from how much weight we gain or lose, to our sex drives and our moods, to how much hair we have. They influence your sleep cycle, your complexion, your reproductive cycle, and your brain functions. When cows are given excessive, unnatural levels of artificial hormones to produce more milk, what effect do you think it might have on you when you drink the milk they produce?

If you've ever taken any sort of a hormone for medical purposes—steroids, birth control pills, cortisone shots—then you know how quickly that small amount of hormone introduced into your body makes dramatic changes. An imbalance of hormones in your body can make you grow hair in unexpected places, create accelerated maturity in children and adolescents, cause you to feel anxious, depressed, angry, or overly emotional, and cause your face to erupt in blemishes.

Antibiotics for Breakfast

Another cause for concern is the antibiotics found in eggs and dairy products, another by-product of factory farming. Over half of the antibiotics produced in the United States go to treat livestock. Certainly, these drugs keep the animals healthy, but are they something you want to be consuming in your food?

The biggest problem with antibiotics is that they're all-purpose bacteria killers. Yes, they kill the viruses and bacteria that can cause disease, but they also kill the good bacteria that we need to keep our body's delicate systems in balance. Good bacteria, like acidophilis and bifidophilis, live in your intestinal tract and on your skin, and they do battle with bad bacteria that can cause you harm.

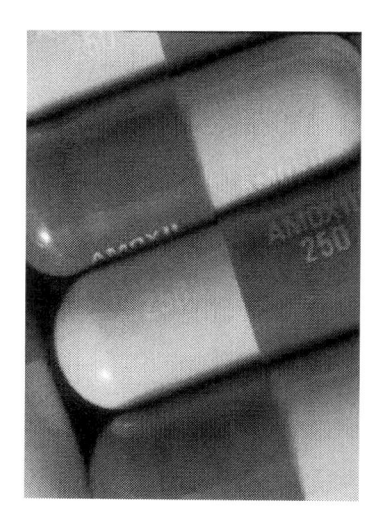

Taking antibiotics on a regular basis, whether by prescription or inadvertently through processed foods, lowers your resistance to bacterial illnesses like salmonella, which is found in small amounts in eggs, poultry, and meat. Normally, your body should be able to fight off the lesser bugs that it ingests but, if you build up a tolerance to antibiotics through constant exposure, your natural immune system is weakened, leaving you more susceptible to illnesses like food poisoning.

On top of that, you may be taking antibiotics prescribed by your doctor, in a carefully measured dose. If you then eat eggs that contain salmonella, it finds no good bacteria waiting to kill it when it hits your small intestine—they've all been done in by the prescription antibiotic. So the salmonella has a nice, warm, moist, antibody-free environment in which to incubate, and you find yourself sick as a dog for a week. Then your doctor prescribes more antibiotics, and the merry-go-round continues.

Dumping the Dairy

Dairy products are included in so many recipes that it may seem like a huge challenge to replace them. Not so! The variety and quality of dairy substitutes has improved greatly in the past decade, and you have a lot of options. If you don't like the taste of one style of nondairy product, just try another; you're bound to find one that works for you.

Cow's milk can be replaced in recipes by rice milk, potato milk, almond milk, or even oat milk. The quantities are the same (1 cup cow's milk = 1 cup rice milk, etc.); the only difference is the taste. Oat milk is very mild, and lacks the sweetness of both cow's milk and other replacements; you may find you prefer it, or you may choose to add more sweetener to compensate. Either way, you have all the control! The nut milks, like almond milk, are quite sweet, and both hemp and rice milk are available with flavors already added. You may find that vanilla rice milk tastes better to you than cow's milk ever did, especially for lightening your coffee or on cereal.

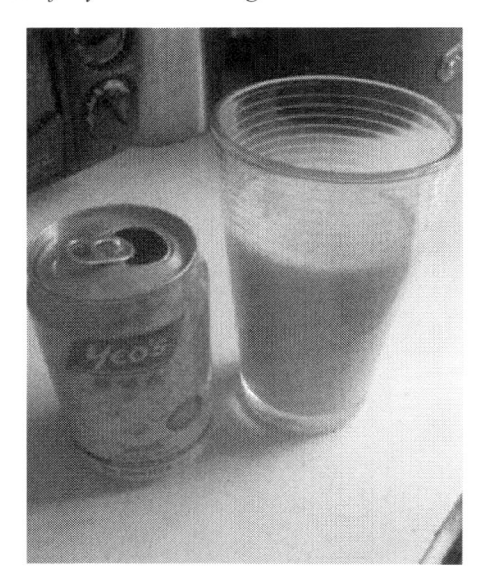

All the milk substitutes can be found in shelf-stable, aseptic boxes at natural foods stores and, increasingly, in supermarkets. This is another advantage over cow's milk— you can save money by purchasing it by the case, if you like, and stock your milk right on the pantry shelf without worrying about it expiring in the fridge (you will want to refrigerate them once opened, however). Rice milk can also be found in powdered form, although you'll probably find that the liquid product tastes better.

Vanilla rice milk works great in desserts; use it to make puddings and custards, on your cereal, in baked foods, and processed in the blender with fresh fruit for smoothies. Plain rice milk works well in savory dishes like casseroles, soups, and sauces. And if you need buttermilk—say, to make buttermilk pancakes—you can create a substitute by adding two teaspoons of vinegar or lemon juice to one cup of rice milk.

Saying Good-bye to Yogurt and Cheese

Yogurt is yummy. Yogurt is healthy. Yogurt is, of course, a dairy product. Because of the active culturing agents in yogurt, it's easier to digest than other types of dairy, but all of the other reasons for giving up this cow's milk product still apply. Fortunately, delicious plain and flavored yogurts are available at your natural foods store. They're cholesterol-free and lower in saturated fat than cow's milk yogurt, so it's even better for you than the dairy version.

Vegan yogurt and sour cream can be used in almost every recipe that would require the use of dairy yogurt. They're great in sauces, dips, and baked foods and can be topped with granola for a quick breakfast. The downside is that they don't work well in hot foods, because they tend to separate when heated.

But what about cheese? Most new vegetarians lean on cheese rather heavily. It provides protein and, honestly, cheese tastes really good. But it's also loaded with cholesterol and saturated fat, and like all dairy products cheese is difficult to digest. If you're ovo-lacto but trying to watch your fat intake, you've probably tried low- or non-fat cheeses, and found them lacking in flavor—they taste awful, don't melt well, and have the texture of a plastic chew toy.

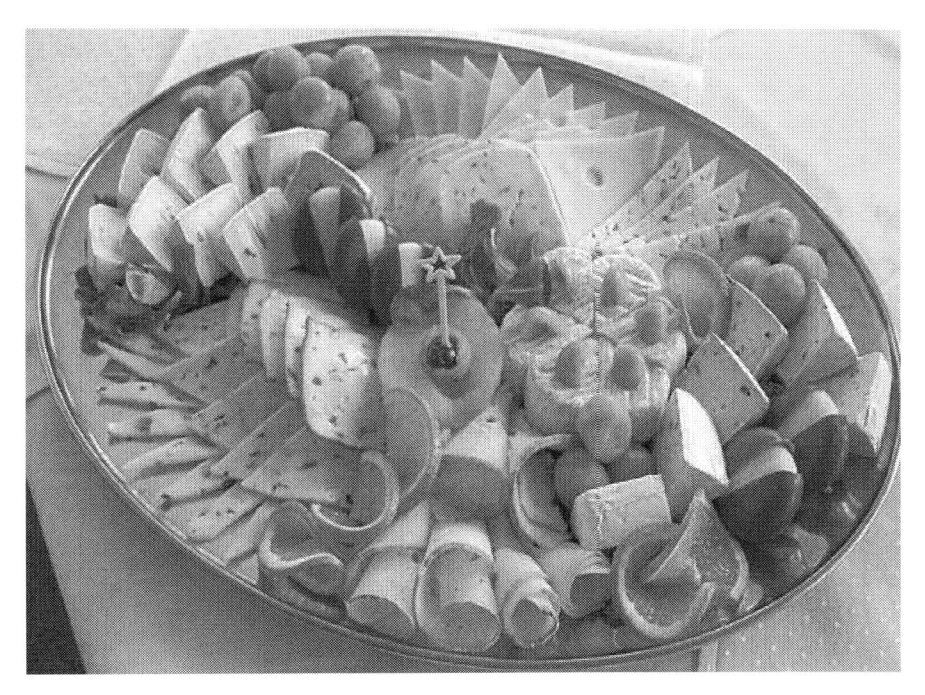

Even if you're not vegan, you should try many varieties of nondairy cheese on the market. Usually nut based, they come in many of the same styles as dairy cheese, like cheddar, mozzarella, jack, or cream cheese. They aren't usually as tasty as the real thing, but they're a close enough approximation, and they work well in sandwiches or recipes.

When cooking with vegan cheese, you'll find that it doesn't melt as well as full-fat dairy cheese (but they're better than nonfat cheese), even though they're fairly high in fat. Some separate a bit when melted, although the oils can be blotted with a paper towel before serving. For Italian dishes like lasagna and manicotti, you can make your own substitute for ricotta or cottage cheese, and if you're going the soy-free route, this can be a bit tough to find. Fortunately, some creativity and research may help. For that cheesy, dry Parmesan taste, try sprinkling some nutritional yeast on spaghetti, casseroles, popcorn, or potatoes; it has a savory taste much like cheese, and it's good for you!

As with milk substitutes, there are many different brands and styles on the market, so, if you don't like the first alternative cheese you try, experiment with a few others until you find one that you like. Remember that most cheese replacements work better as ingredients in recipes and sandwiches than eaten on their own. But there are so many healthy snacks that you can munch on, you don't need to eat straight cheese, anyway.

Who's Got the Butter?

That vegetable-based margarine in your grocer's cold case isn't dairy-free. It's made with casein, a milk protein, and probably has other animal products in it, too. If you're ovo-lacto, you may not care too much, but if you're vegan, there's special margarine available at your natural foods store.

For most purposes, look to olive oil. Even nonvegetarians are better off stepping away from butter because of its high cholesterol and steering clear of margarine because of the trans fats. Margarine, made from vegetable oil, is semi-solid because of the way it's produced; the molecular composition of the fats are altered to create *trans fatty acids*, making them solid enough to spread on bread or form into sticks for commercial sale. While many people long assumed that margarine was healthier than butter because of its low cholesterol and vegetable origins, scientists now know that trans fats are even more dangerous than the saturated fat of butter and can lead to clogged arteries and heart disease.

Olive oil is good for you. Studies into the health benefits of olive oil have found that it can actually reduce blood cholesterol levels, thus lowering the risk of coronary heart disease. In one study, the subjects' risks of fatal heart attacks were cut 50 percent in two to four years when they started eating the so-called Mediterranean diet—a diet which, interestingly, prescribes increased consumption of fruits, vegetables, and whole grains, limited animal foods, and the use of olive oil as the main source of dietary fat.

In addition, a 2006 study at the Monell Chemical Senses Center in Philadelphia found that olive oil has anti-inflammatory qualities. The active ingredient in olives and olive oil has a similar effect on the body as aspirin and ibuprofen! So use more olive oil, feel better, and be healthier!

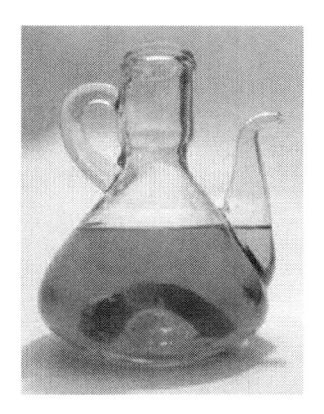

CHAPTER 16

Special Needs
How to Live a Meatless Life and Still Make Your Doctor (or Coach) Happy

If you have an ongoing health concern like diabetes, if you're pregnant (or trying to conceive), or if you're an athlete in training for a sport, you naturally have concerns about whether a vegetarian diet is your best option. The answer is yes—if you're eating enough of the right foods. Vegetarianism is great for keeping blood sugar under control and getting the body in peak shape, whether you hope to run a marathon or have a baby.

Doing Vegetarianism as a Diabetic

For diabetics, diet is the first line of defense, literally the difference between life and death. Left untreated, diabetes can cause blindness, kidney failure, and even loss of the hands and feet, and it affects people of all ages. If you're a diabetic, your doctor has already told you that your diet is the single most important way you can manage your diabetes. A low-fat, high-carbohydrate, and high-fiber vegetarian diet is an excellent option.

Worldwide, over thirty million people suffer from diabetes. Essentially, the condition is one in which the body is unable to process nutrients efficiently. In a normal body, the food we eat is converted to usable energy in the form of glucose, a sugar that's carried by the blood to all of our various functions with the help of the hormone insulin. Diabetics, however, have an imbalance of insulin—either too little or none at all—which means that the body has difficulty converting blood sugar to usable energy. This means that the glucose remains, unconverted, in the bloodstream and never gets where it's needed. This leads to fatigue, muscle pain, loss of concentration and coordination, and blurry vision. When someone has a hypoglycemic episode, that's what's going on—the amount of usable sugars in their bloodstream is too low. In extreme cases this can lead to the person lapsing into a coma, or even dying.

As a matter of controlling their blood sugar, diabetics have to keep a close eye on their diet, eating a wide variety of foods and making sure they sit down to regular meals. Carbohydrates must be watched carefully. At least half of the recommended diabetic diet must include complex carbohydrates from sources like baked potatoes, whole-grain breads, vegetables, and legumes. Sounds like a vegetarian diet, doesn't it?

In fact, the vegetarian diet is so good for diabetics that some vegetarian diabetics can transition off medication, including many who previously had to inject insulin. For optimum result, eat organic raw vegan diet, there is a documentary on this, at www.rawfor30days.com that actually reverses diabetes. If you have diabetes, or know someone that does, pls take a look on the site.

Adding a Third Vegetarian to the Family

If you're hoping to get pregnant, both you and your doctor want you to be in the best possible condition to insure that both you and your baby are healthy. Eating well is important before and during pregnancy. And the more of a head start you can get on good health before you conceive, the better.

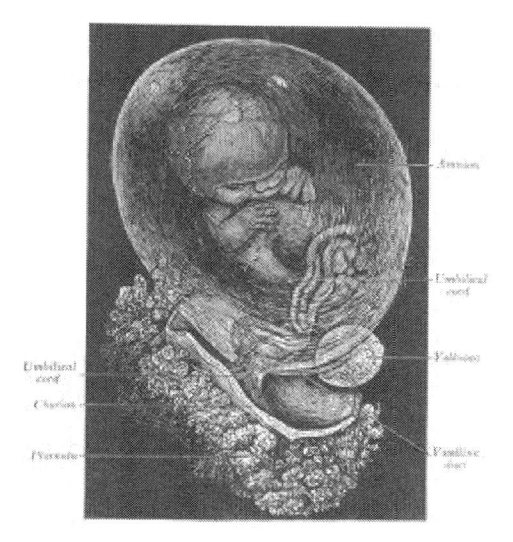

Vegetarians may eat a healthier diet than omnivores, but you'll still need to follow the same advice as nonvegetarians in many respects. Take a daily multivitamin and mineral supplement for several months before you get pregnant, and make sure it offers plenty of B1 of the spine and brain. Get plenty of physical activity and drink lots of water; avoid alcohol, tobacco, and caffeine. Eat nutritious foods and cut back or eliminate junk food and refined sugar.

As a vegetarian, you'll probably be in better shape and closer to your ideal weight than if you were eating meat. Now that you're avoiding animal foods, you'll also have a strong immune system which you'll pass on to your baby. Just make sure that you're getting plenty of iron. Many women begin pregnancy deficient in iron, and as your body grows and you store more blood to nourish your baby, you don't want to risk becoming anemic.

Enough Protein for Two

Once you've conceived, and you know that you're carrying a child, you'll probably start to worry about getting all the nutrients you need for you and your baby. But protein really isn't your biggest concern. As we've already noted, most people already eat too much protein. If you're eating a healthy diet consisting of a variety of foods, you're probably getting plenty of protein from whole grains, beans, legumes, and either dairy or rice milk.

A greater concern is that you get enough omega-3 fatty acids—a nutrient that plays an important role in brain function and development—as well as calcium, folic acid, iron, zinc, and vitamins B12 and D. If you're a pesco vegetarian (one who eats fish), you can get plenty of omega-3s by eating fatty fish like salmon. If you don't eat fish, add ground flaxseed (found at natural food stores or your supermarket) to your meals, or take a supplement. The rest of the important nutrients should be plentiful, if you follow some simple recommendations:

Eat four servings of cooked dried beans and peas each day; they're full of zinc, iron, and protein. Munch on nuts and seeds, but be careful of eating too much fat.

Include four servings of calcium-rich foods. Read labels on dairy and milk substitutes, and try to get 30 percent of the RDA of calcium—that's 300 mg of calcium per serving. Use rice milks that are fortified with vitamin D, which helps your body process calcium.

Eat from five to seven servings of vegetables and three to five servings of fresh fruit each day, for energy, vitamins, fiber, and antioxidants.

Include six to eleven servings of whole grains, like bread, cereal, brown rice, and oatmeal.

Get your vitamin B12 by eating at least one serving each day of B12-rich foods like milk, fortified rice milk, miso, and tempeh.

If you find yourself eating too little and you need to consume more calories, shakes and smoothies are tasty, easy to digest, and full of nutrients.

High Performance from Plant Foods

If you actively train for a sport, you've probably already heard that you can't reach top performance on a vegetarian diet—and a vegan diet, well, that's right out! But it's not. Many world-class athletes are vegetarians, including some very famous names. Baseball legend Hank

Aaron, exercise guru Jack LaLanne, professional skateboarder Steve Berra, football player Joe Namath, three-time Ironman champion Ruth Heidrish, Olympic track star Carl Lewis, and tennis greats Billie Jean King and Martina Navratilova are among thousands of professional athletes who built their bodies on vegetarian and vegan diets.

Athletes are among the few vegetarians that actually need to worry about getting enough protein in their diets. When animal products are removed from the diet, considerably less protein is being consumed, and a highly active body requires more protein than that of the average person. When there's too little dietary protein, carbohydrates enter the bloodstream faster, causing insulin levels to rise quickly, and then plunge a short time later. This is the dreaded sugar crash that we've all experienced, and it's a killer for athletes who depend on a steady supply of usable energy. Additional protein in the diet balances the carbohydrates, heading off the sugar crash by releasing energy into the bloodstream at a more efficient rate.

Protein is also important to athletes as it's used to rebuild muscle tissue during training. The way in which muscles are grown and strengthened is an ongoing process of breaking down tissue and then building them back up again. Without enough protein, the taxed muscles won't rebuild themselves.

It's a simple matter to add protein to a vegetarian diet. You've already read about the amazing variety of plant foods that provide adequate protein. Adding one or two protein-rich snacks each day can boost your protein intake by ten to twenty-five grams. A cup of vegetarian chili over rice, a bowl of whole-grain cereal with hemp milk, a whole-wheat roll with peanut butter, a large baked potato, and a cup of soup are all great protein-rich snacks.

Scientists, physicians, and sports trainers all know that a high-carbohydrate diet is best for athletes, as the carbs provide necessary energy and stamina. Sugar that's stored in the muscles for their use is called "glycogen," and your body uses these stored sugars when performing both endurance activities like running, swimming, and biking, and lower-intensity activities like sprinting, skiing, and snowboarding. The vegetarian diet, with its emphasis on whole grains, legumes, fruit, and vegetables, offers the necessary high intake of carbohydrate.

A vegetarian diet should provide all the vitamins and minerals that athletes require, but if you're training hard, you should make sure you eat enough foods that provide vital nutrients like iron, zinc (found in fortified breakfast cereals, legumes, nuts, and seeds), and vitamin C to enhance the absorption of iron.

There is some concern that the vegetarian or vegan diet puts female athletes at a higher risk for amenorrhea (irregular menstrual cycles) and osteoporosis. Some studies have associated high-fiber, low-fat vegetarian diets combined with extremely high levels of exercise with reduced estrogen levels. The consensus among scientists, though, is that the fault lies in low-energy intake—not consuming enough calories—rather than in the vegetarian diet. These same studies have found that female athletes have normal menstrual cycles when they increase their caloric intake.

What to Eat on Game Day

If you already consume a good amount of carbohydrates, then you are on the right track. Here are some more tips to use on game day so that you will be able to perform at a highly competitive level:

Easy digestion. In the last few hours before the actual event or game, eat foods that are easily digested through the body. This is where you will want to eat less fat and protein. Fat and protein take a long time to digest, and you don't want food sitting in the pit of your stomach right before the event or game. You want the food to be at that point in your intestines where nutrients are easily absorbed and can provide you with bursts of energy. Eat fruits, vegetables, and grains leading up to the game or event, and you'll have an amazing performance!

Avoiding dehydration. Dehydration is an athlete's worst enemy. The last thing you want to do is cramp up during a game or event. Avoid any and all foods that contain salt, and drink lots of water. Also avoid foods that are high in fiber. They will absorb the water in your body and possibly cause stomach cramps and/or diarrhea.

Rule of thumb. Before any athletic event or game, you want to give yourself one hour for every two hundred calories you consume. For example, if you eat a meal containing six hundred calories, you'll want to eat it three hours before the actual event.

What to Eat After the Game

Replenishing your body after an athletic event is extremely important. Once the game or event is over, you can return your focus to protein in order to reenergize and feed your muscles. Your body will need to restock its supply of amino acids, fluids, and liver glycogen. That is why protein bars or shakes with a high amount of calories and carbohydrates are important to eat immediately after a game. Fluids are important too, which is why you see a lot of athletes drinking water or Gatorade. The sooner you replenish your body with fluids and nutrients, the sooner your body will recover from the game or event. Then you can work on getting ready for your next competition.

The Aging Vegetarian

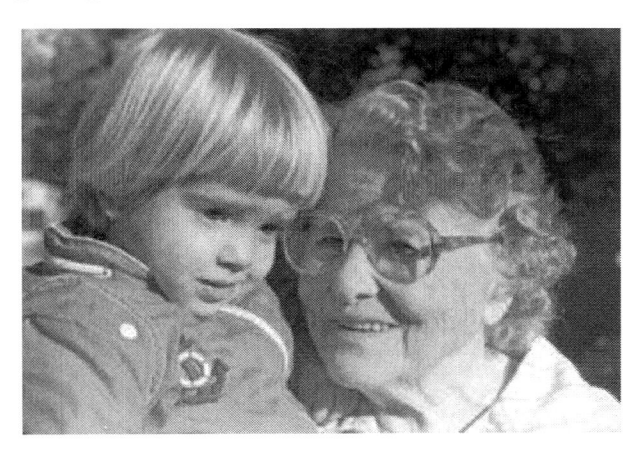

Gerontology—the study of old age and aging—is a relatively new science, and little is known about the specific nutritional needs of older people as compared to that of children and younger adults. Many people live out their seniority with vigor, but even they notice that certain health problems can increase as they age. One thing that scientists know is that much of how we age is genetic. There are certainly patterns to how all humans change as they age, but those changes come at a different pace for different people. Some of that difference is genetic, and some of it is due to diet and lifestyle.

As we've already discussed, the right diet can improve your health and allow you to live longer. Research into the health and longevity of vegetarians has shown that those who eat a vegetarian diet that's lower in calories, saturated fat, and protein, and higher in fiber and phytochemicals suffer from less obesity, heart disease, high blood pressure, diabetes, and vulnerability to some forms of cancer than nonvegetarians—and they tend to live longer, too.

Good eating habits in the years that lead up to old age will not only help your current health but will help to minimize the various ailments that plague the elderly. Your genes will play a part in how you age. But a healthy vegetarian diet will help, no matter what genetic cards you've drawn.

One thing that researchers agree upon is that older adults need less calories as they age. Part of that is due to the inevitable decline in the rate of metabolism. Like it or not, your metabolism will slow as you age, meaning you will need to consume less energy to keep your body functioning. You'll also, in most cases, become less physically active—another reason you'll need less calories. And yet, you'll still need the same amount of various nutrients that you always did; in some cases, you'll need more.

As people age, it becomes more likely that specific medical problems will require a special diet. Those with diabetes, high blood pressure, and heart disease will need to plan their diets according to their physician's recommendations. Most conditions, however, benefit from a diet that's high in fiber from whole grains, fruits, and vegetables, and low in animal products, and we already know that a vegetarian lifestyle can help to keep blood sugar levels in check. If you follow a special diet, consult with a nutritionist or dietitian for help with vegetarian meal planning.

You may also be hoping that a healthier diet will help with arthritis. Yes, it is does! In fact, because you don't consume animal proteins anymore, it's much harder to get it. A low-fat vegetarian diet will help you maintain optimum weight, which has been proven to lessen or even prevent some symptoms of arthritis.

There are a number of factors that can affect the eating habits of older adults. Sometimes money plays a part. Many elderly people are on tight budgets, and they don't get proper nutrition because of financial stress. Others find it difficult to tolerate a lot of foods as they age, or they're unable to shop and cook for themselves, so their diet suffers. Older people with diabetes or high blood pressure have to modify their diets significantly, and sometimes there are problems with chewing or swallowing that keep them from eating as much as they should.

The most important thing to remember as you age—and this applies to anyone who is over 40 and notices their metabolism slowing down—is that you need to get as much nutrition from the food you eat as possible while keeping an eye on caloric intake. That means cutting out the empty calories that come from junk foods—consuming less sweets, chips, soft drinks, and alcohol—while eating more nutrient-dense foods that give you real bang for your caloric buck.

The basic recommendations for all adults are even more important for older people. In a nutshell:

>Limit your intake of:
>
>Sweets
>Regular coffee and tea
>Greasy or fatty foods
>Alcohol
>Oil, margarine, and junk foods
>Other added fat
>Salt
>
>Eat plenty of:
>
>Fruits
>Whole-grain breads and cereals
>Vegetables
>Drink plenty of fluids, especially water

Special Problems of Older Adults

The biggest source of discomfort in older adults is digestive problems. Unfortunately, this often causes people to avoid foods that are rich in nutrients that they need—flatulence, for example, may inspire them to cut out foods like beans and cabbage, both of which are rich in vitamins, minerals, and fiber. Sometimes, the answer is to add other foods to the diet to compensate.

Let's look at some common problems that affect us as we age:

Constipation is a common complaint, usually caused by not drinking enough fluids and by not eating enough fiber. Some medications, like antacids made with aluminum hydroxide or calcium carbonate, can increase the risk of constipation, and habitual use of laxatives actually makes the problem worse. The first step in avoiding constipation is to eat a diet that includes lots of whole-grain breads and cereals, and plenty of vegetables and fruits. Many people find that eating dried fruits like prunes or figs helps, as they have a natural laxative effect for many people (your grandpa drank all that prune juice for a reason). Make sure you drink plenty of fluids, especially water, and limit foods that are high in fat, including high-fat dairy products, oils, margarine, and fried foods. Regular exercise helps too.

Gas and heartburn often plague older adults, especially after eating. The symptoms are both uncomfortable and embarrassing—belching, intestinal gas or flatulence, bloating, and a burning sensation in the stomach and chest. They're caused by a number of different things, including overeating, eating too many high-fat foods, and drinking alcohol or carbonated beverages. Lying down to rest right after eating and taking certain drugs—including aspirin—can contribute to the problem too. Eating a high-fiber diet often works, although sometimes the symptoms return when the body adjusts to the increased fiber intake. To battle indigestion, try eating smaller, more frequent meals instead of one or two larger meals. Eat slowly and chew food thoroughly before swallowing. As with constipation, regular exercise can help minimize problems with gas.

Chewing and swallowing problems are an unfortunate way of life for many older adults. Raw foods are good, but not everybody can eat it all the time, so cooking vegetables and fruits may be necessary, even though the foods lose some of their nutrient value in the process. Cutting your food into smaller pieces and taking extra time to chew by not rushing meals may also be helpful. If you wear dentures, check with your dentist to make sure that you have the proper fit; our mouths change as we age, and they may need to be replaced. Make sure to drink plenty of fluids, especially water, and keep it on hand during meals—some medications contribute to dry mouth and could be adding to the problem.

Loss of appetite is a common problem for the elderly, and it's sometimes caused by depression. Depression is common in older people, because of changes in their living conditions, the loss of beloved companions, side effects of some medications, and difficulty in caring for themselves. Eating a number of small meals throughout the day may help, and it's also good to seek out opportunities to socialize over meals. A nearby senior center probably offers regular meals, and you can discuss your vegetarian needs with their dietitian. You can also contact your local vegetarian groups and ask if they sponsor restaurant outings or potluck dinners, which can give you the chance to get out, have a nice meal with good company, and make some new friends!

Meal Planning for Older Adults

Seniors often find that meal planning is a challenge, especially if it's difficult for them to shop and cook. Arthritis can make it tough to manage a trip through the grocery store, open bottles, or handle cooking utensils. Impaired eyesight may make it difficult to drive to the store and read food labels or package instructions, and it's sometimes hard to be motivated to cook when you're only making meals for yourself.

If this applies to you, you'll need to plan meals that are simple, quick, and easy to prepare. Ready-to-eat breakfast cereals are a great snack or easy meal, and hot cereals like oatmeal can be cooked in a microwave in just a manner of minutes. Canned fruits and vegetables have a long shelf life, and will keep for months in the pantry. Whole-grain breads, muffins, tortillas, and bagels can be stored in the freezer, so you can thaw just enough for one meal at a time. Also stick your pantry with frozen vegetables, whole-grain crackers, peanut or almond butter, canned beans, and shelf-stable cartons of rice milk.

If you're able to cook, make a full recipe that normally serves six or eight people and then freeze individual servings to be eaten later. Veggie lasagna, casseroles, cheese enchiladas, vegetarian chili, whole-grain cookies, and muffins or pancakes all freeze well, and can be reheated as needed for a quick meal.

CHAPTER 17

Veggies for Kids
How to Raise a Happy, Healthy Vegetarian Child

We all start out life as lacto-vegetarians. Out first food is our mothers' milk, full of all the nutrients we need. Infant formula, the alternative to breast milk, is made as close as possible to that of mother's milk, and it's all we require or should eat for the first four to six months of life. The good news is, if you're a vegetarian, your breast milk is superior to that of nonvegetarian mothers because you're not passing on any of the antibiotics, pesticides, or other contaminants that you would if you were eating meat. (And if you're a vegan and you breast-feed, your child is still a vegan, too; breast milk is a natural food for humans while cow's milk is not).

Whether or not you breastfeed is entirely your decision, but, for most babies, breast milk is the optimal food. In addition to the sugars and other nutrients, scientists believe that there are other, as yet unidentified, substances in breast milk that make it superior to infant formula. Should you decide not to breast-feed, choose a vegetarian formula—although soy is less likely to cause allergies than cow's-milk-based formulas, it's not designed to meet their nutritional needs. It is my recommendation that you avoid using soy milk altogether.

Cow's milk should never be fed to babies under one year old, as it can cause intestinal bleeding and lead to anemia. Also, studies have shown a link between infants drinking cow's milk and their increased risk to become diabetic later in life.

Meat-free Infants

At the four-to-six-month mark, it's time to introduce your baby to solid foods. The timing varies from baby to baby. When your child reaches thirteen pounds or double his birth weight, he may want to breast-feed eight times or more during a twenty-four-hour period, and when he takes a quart or more of a formula per day and still act hungry, it's time to transition to solid foods.

You'll want to introduce solid foods slowly, so that their systems can get used to the change in diet. Start with cooked grains. Rice cereal is best, as almost every baby can digest it easily, and it is unlikely to cause an allergic reaction. Once your baby eats cooked cereal, begin to slowly introduce other foods. You can buy commercial baby foods or puree your own fruits and vegetables in a blender. If you buy prepared foods, buy ones that are free from added sugars, preservatives, and any other additives that your baby doesn't need. Start with raw, mashed fruits and move on to cooked vegetables like mashed sweet potatoes. It's smart to introduce new foods one at a time, so, if your baby has sensitivity to a food, you can easily identify it.

When your child starts teething (somewhere between twelve and twenty-four months), they can move on to foods that need to be chewed. Raw vegetables can be introduced then, starting with veggies that are easy to chew and unlikely to present a choking hazard. When giving babies finger foods, take care that the foods aren't too hard, large, sharp, or round. Good choices are carrot sticks, lettuce, and other leafy green vegetables, and lightly blanched and cooled broccoli. As long as it's safe for the baby to chew, vegetables that adults eat are fine for a child.

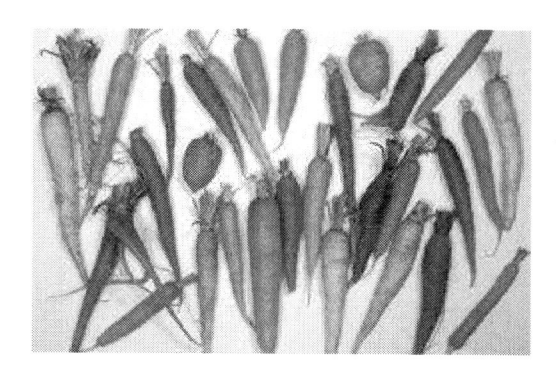

Follow the same feeding schedules and advice that you would for any other baby, except for not feeding them meat. Adapt the guidelines in the baby books to the vegetarian diet. Just make sure that you don't let other people convince you that you should be allowing your baby to drink cow's milk. Once your child is old enough to transition off formula, you can give him water, regular or flavored rice milk, juice, or any other nutritious liquid.

At seven to ten months, start introducing high-protein legumes to the baby's diet. Add about two servings per day, about a half-ounce per serving. Most babies are very fond of lentils, which can be cooked until fairly soft and have a pleasant, bland flavor. Nut butters should not be fed until after twelve months.

Toddler Time

As you ease into the toddler/preschooler years (ages one to four), you can start offering your child some vegetarian versions of classic kids' favorites. Vegetarian and vegan children are just like any other kids, They'll be a bit fussy sometimes, but there are a wide variety of nutritious foods that children universally enjoy:

> Spaghetti with meatless sauce
> Peanut butter and jelly sandwiches
> Baked French fries with ketchup
> Veggie burgers, hot dogs, and sandwich slices
> Whole wheat bread and rolls
> Grilled soy-free cheese sandwiches
> Veggie pizzas with soy-free cheese
> Pancakes or waffles, with fruit or maple syrup
> Vegetable soup
> Baked potatoes with nondairy sour cream
> Rice and beans
> Spinach lasagna
> Calcium-fortified rice milk and orange juice
> Cold cereal with vanilla rice milk
> Chicken-free nuggets (vegetarian nuggets that taste just like breaded chicken)

Snacks:

>Fruit, cut up into bite-sized pieces
>Raisins and banana chips
>Trail mix
>Applesauce
>Fruit smoothies
>Popcorn
>Vegan cakes, cookies, and other baked foods

Vegetarian diets feature a lot of bulky, filling plant foods, and since small children have equally small stomachs, they sometimes don't get all the calories they require. Make sure to include a lot of calorie-dense foods in your child's diet so that they get all the energy their growing bodies require—for example, you can add avocado, which is calorie-dense and full of good fats, to sandwiches. Peanut and almond butters are excellent sources of calories for kids too.

Very young children also need to eat more than three meals each day. So be generous with the snacks featuring grains, fruits, and vegetables to add lots of necessary nutrients to their diet. Don't worry about a vegetarian diet affecting your child's growth. A 1989 study of children living in a vegan community in Tennessee found that while they were slightly shorter than average at age one to three, they caught up by age ten, when they were actually taller than average, and weighed slightly less than children raised on an omnivorous diet.

Defeating the Threat of Childhood Obesity

Childhood obesity has ballooned (excuse the pun) to the point where expert nutritionists and numerous doctors now classify it as a threatening disease. The obesity problem is a direct result of everyday diets consisting of soda, junk food, fast food, and sugar-rich foods. Lack of consistent physical activity is also a major contributing factor. Sedentary lifestyles, where more time is spent playing video games, watching television, or sitting in front of the computer, have become commonplace.

The solution starts at home. You can make a difference in your children's lives simply by introducing a vegetarian diet. It has been proven that children who eat less meat and more fiber-rich fruits and vegetables are more likely to maintain a normal body weight. Eating less sugar, less sodium, and less saturated fat as a child will enable them to develop healthy bodies as they grow older. You can also encourage your children to be active. Limit their television time and computer use. Get them outside on the weekends for hikes, walks, and bike rides. You'll be amazed at the difference, not only in their weight but also in their attitude!

School-age Vegetarians

While most vegetarian children have traditionally been raised as such since birth, more and more kids as young as eight or nine are choosing the lifestyle for themselves. This is great! And despite concerns, they usually don't find themselves suffering socially because of it. A lot of children have to avoid various foods, like dairy, nuts, and chocolate, due to allergies, and vegetarian/vegan kids are no different.

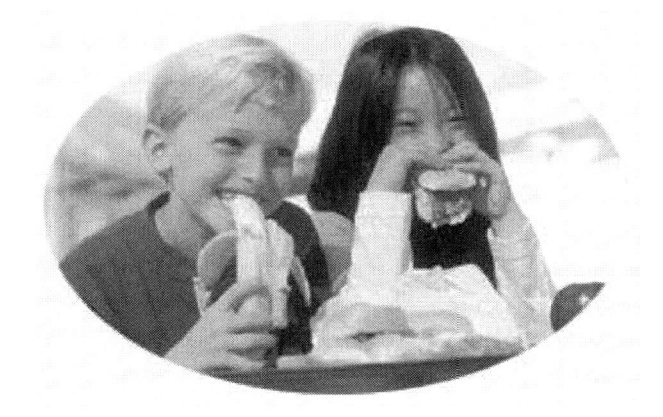

You'll probably have to provide them with snacks and lunches from home, as school menus usually offer few vegetarian choices—although they may offer juice, vegetables, and fruits, dairy-free breads, baked potatoes, and even bean burritos. If your child's school offers a weekly menu, you can plan ahead of time, discussing with your child what they will or won't eat, and what you can supplement from home. This is also a great opportunity to get your child involved in making responsible food choices!

During the teen years, a lot of kids choose vegetarian diets themselves for moral and ethical reasons. This is terrific, but teenagers are still teenagers whether they eat meat or not. You'll soon find your teen gravitating toward cookies, chips, French fries, and candy, and away from salads and raw vegetables. Work with your child, and patiently try to get them to eat less empty calories and more nutrient-dense foods.

It's normal for teenagers to be conscious of their weight, even though it may not be healthy. Because of the images and messages portrayed in the media, most girls strive to be thinner while most boys want to achieve muscle mass and become larger. You can help give girls a better outlook on the reasons to be leaner by incorporating fresh fruits, vegetables, whole grains, and plant-based foods into their diet. Help them realize that a person's weight shouldn't be viewed from an image perspective, but rather a healthy, physical perspective. As for boys who want to gain weight, teach them to do it properly. Provide them with protein shakes and healthy snacks between meals. Give them larger portions of good foods instead of letting them pile on empty calories. Body image and daily diets go hand in hand. You can easily influence your child's outlook on weight in a positive way through the principles of vegetarianism.

Teens with eating disorders often latch onto a vegan diet as a socially acceptable way to control their food and not eat, so if your child is losing a great deal of weight and shows other signs of anorexia or bulimia, deal immediately with the problem. Vegan diets do not lead to eating disorders; it's a serious mental health problem that may need professional intervention. If your teen appears to be seriously underweight, first talk to them about their diet and work with them to make changes so that they're getting the nutrition they need. But if the problem persists and you suspect your child has an eating disorder, seek professional help.

Teen athletes who eat a vegetarian diet need a decent amount of protein and other nutrients to stay active and competitive. It's important to remember that teens need certain nutrients more than adults do because their body is in a stage of growth and development. An active teen could increase the need for these nutrients even further. Make sure that their caloric intake is based on good and wholesome foods instead of high-sugar foods. They'll be able to take in all the nutrients they need as well as a sufficient amount of calories to burn for energy.

Nutrition for all ages

Because children are growing—and growing rapidly—they need a lot of nutrients to fuel their growth. Calcium is especially important, as bones are growing during this period. So make sure they eat plenty of leafy green vegetables and legumes and drink calcium-fortified orange juice. Calcium-rich foods are usually full of iron, too, which is great because children need a lot of iron; make sure they also get plenty of vitamin C to help absorb the iron.

The vitamin family should be represented too. If they're eating a variety of foods, they should be getting enough B12 and D, but if you're concerned about their nutrient consumption, there are vegan multivitamins for children available at your natural foods store.

Kids are notoriously fussy, but when presented with a variety of tasty, appealing, and convenient foods, they'll have no trouble enjoying a vegetarian diet. By keeping your cupboards free of empty-calorie foods and providing an array of healthful snacks—like, baby carrots, fresh fruit, hummus, whole-wheat crackers, and whole-grain breads—you'll encourage your kids to eat healthy foods and set the stage for their healthy adult diets.

And, of course, you can do your part to make them feel good about their vegetarian lifestyle by setting a good example with your own eating habits. That means making delicious meals for the entire family and turning mealtime into a pleasant, bonding experience. Try not to nag them about their food choices; they're kids, and they're still learning about what they like to eat. If your shelves are full of healthy, tasty foods, that's the first thing they'll grab when they get hungry. And if you raise them to enjoy fresh fruit, vegetables, and whole grains as toddlers, they're less likely to go overboard on junk foods when they hit their teens.

CHAPTER 18

The Social Vegetarian Connecting with Meat Eaters and Others at Work and at Play

People are now less inclined to look down their noses at vegetarians than in the past, but there are still social challenges to living a vegetarian life. Some people will believe that you're making an in-your-face political choice and will have a negative reaction for no good reason. A lot of people will wonder if you've gone all hippy-dippy, patchouli-scented goofball on them, and treat you with condescension and scorn. Even the most supportive of friends will misunderstand what vegetarian means and offer you fish or eggs without ever asking you for the particulars of your diet. And you're going to have to take this all with good humor and flexibility. The level of acceptance you find depends, of course, on where you live, where you work, and what sort of people you hang out with. But even in the most accepting of environments, you're going to have challenges.

Explaining Yourself—Even though You Shouldn't Have to

As we've discussed, you'll need a supply of quick, polite answers to handle the questions people will have about your diet. Don't get cranky. Sure, they're nosy, but isn't it nice that they want to know more about vegetarianism? If you already know what to say, it'll be easy to give them an answer without turning the conversation into a lengthy debate. Some of the most common questions you'll field are the same ones you had when you first started out—except now you know the answers:

> Why are you a vegetarian?
> If you don't eat meat, how do you get enough protein?
> Can you eat chicken? How about fish?
> Is this some sort of a religious thing?
> Is it hard to never eat meat?
> Why do you wear leather shoes if you won't eat animals?
> Isn't vegetarian food boring?
> Can you eat at McDonald's?
>
> If you already know the answers, you won't mind the questions so much!

Dining Gracefully with Nonvegetarians

Dinner parties—both attending them and hosting them—can be problematic for people on special diets. If you're the host, you can make sure that you have a tempting variety of delicious foods and dazzle your guests with such tasty choices that they'd be foolish to miss the meat. But what if you're the guest?

Often, even if your hosts know that you're vegetarian, they may not know how to feed you. They may think that by serving grilled salmon instead of meat loaf they're offering a vegetarian-friendly entree. Or you may end up in a situation where your hosts simply have no idea of what your needs are.

In those cases, you need to make the best of things. Etiquette is, fundamentally, about behaving well under challenging circumstances. If all there is on the table that you can eat is bread and salad, do so. And, if you're questioned, smile and say that they're so delicious that you're happy to enjoy them. Even if it's disappointing, remember that it's just for one meal; chat with your tablemates, enjoy the company, and have a good time anyway!

If there's absolutely nothing on the menu that you can eat, or your hostess sits a plate of animal food in front of you, do what children do—squish things around and mess up your plate. Hide the meat under some lettuce, and leave some empty space so it looks like you ate something. If the conversation is compelling, most people won't notice how much you did, or didn't, eat. (But don't eat it, no matter what.)

Whatever happens, don't make an issue of your diet. To be blunt, no one is really interested in what you can't eat, and it's considered rude to draw all of the conversation to yourself in such a manner anyway. If someone asks, just say that you're a vegetarian and steer the conversation to something else.

If you're headed to a big social event like a wedding or a family dinner, and you think there might be challenges finding something to eat, then eat a light meal before you leave the house. Even under the worst circumstances, there will be something for you to snack on, but you won't be suffering from hunger pangs throughout the evening.

Being a Great, Vegetarian Hostess

Part of being a terrific host is anticipating your guests' needs. Think about how you'd like to be treated when you go to dinner at a friend's home. How about offering the same courtesy to them? When you invite guests to dinner, ask them if they have special dietary needs, or if there's anything they absolutely hate. You'll be surprised at what people have to say—some may be allergic to bell peppers, or peanuts, or dairy. If you accommodate their needs that same way you'd like yours accommodated in a similar situation, you can make them feel extra welcome in your home.

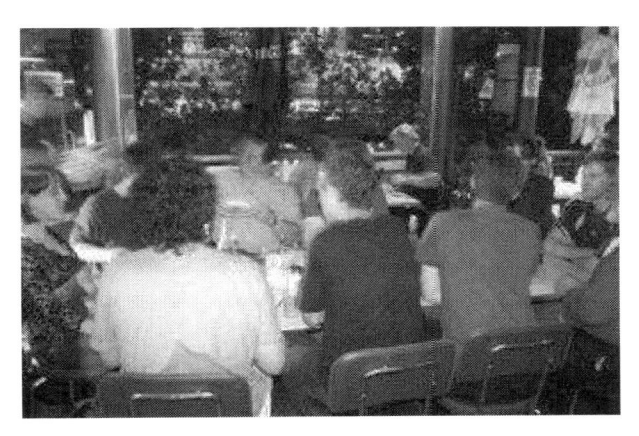

One sure way to make everyone happy is to serve a variety of different dishes buffet style, allowing guests to fill their plates only with what they want. It helps them to feel comfortable if they don't want to eat something—no one will be looking at their plate and wondering why there's still food there—and it'll save you the effort of serving, so you have more time to enjoy your guests.

Only serve meat if you genuinely feel comfortable doing so. Some people will cook a chicken or fish dish for guests, but not partake of it themselves. If you're happy doing this, then go ahead. But if you aren't, then make them the best vegetarian meal they've ever tasted, and show them how delicious eating meat-free can be!

You can also put some extra effort into how you present the meal. For example, a simple garnish (an orange slice or a piece of cilantro) can add a little something to any plate. Also, rid the room of any distractions. Turn off the television, put on some dinner music, add some soft lighting, place some fresh flowers on the table, and you've got the perfect atmosphere for a fantastic vegetarian meal with family and/or friends!

Happy holidays, vegetarian style

Hosting holiday parties or dinners for family and friends can be quite an undertaking. But hosting holiday parties or dinners as a vegetarian can be another experience altogether. You may be a bit apprehensive about what to make, especially as a new vegetarian, because you don't want to revert back to the old way of eating. Planning a brand-new vegetarian menu that will be good for you and make your guests happy isn't as difficult as you may think!

When it comes to Thanksgiving, people expect turkey. When it comes to Easter, people expect ham. This is where a bit of creativity comes in. You can make these traditional holiday items with a vegetarian twist. All you need is an open mind, some willing guests, and some commonsense.

Take Thanksgiving for instance. What do nonvegetarians usually indulge in on this traditional holiday? Isn't it typically some turkey, pumpkin pie, stuffing, sweet potatoes, and some bean casserole of some kind? All of these traditional Thanksgiving dishes can be made vegetarian style. Instead of a turkey, serve up a vegan nut roast. Some vegetarians even opt to serve a different entrée other than turkey, like stuffed shells or vegetable lasagna. As for the side dishes, you can easily substitute a vegetarian casserole or make a hearty leafy-green salad. Macaroni and cheese makes a great side dish as well, unless you're a vegan. Never be afraid to experiment with pumpkin dishes as well. Pumpkin soup, or tiny individually stuffed pumpkins make a great side dish or appetizer. The grand finale, or the pumpkin pie, can also be made vegetarian style. Use rice milk instead of milk or eggs for the actual filling. Your guests probably won't even notice the difference.

Even with traditional holiday meals, there are no absolute rules to follow. If your family and friends are open to trying new dishes, take advantage of the opportunity. Chances are they will feel much lighter and healthier after eating a vegetarian Thanksgiving meal instead of a meat-filled one. They won't be suffering from a turkey-induced coma or feel bloated and uncomfortable, and they will *thank you* for it!

Meat and the Vegetarian Single

If you're single and dating, you've probably already figured out that it's a special sort of challenge. Do you date people who eat meat? Or are you only interested in dating other vegetarians?

Vegetarian singles that choose to date those who aren't vegetarian or vegan may find themselves at a disadvantage. Many vegetarians can't stand to watch people eat meat, and going out to dinner with a potential romantic partner who's chewing on a big, rare steak is a disaster waiting to happen. Dating nonvegetarians can be stressful for vegetarians—after all, you may find yourself repulsed at the thought of kissing someone who just ate a cheeseburger!

On the other hand, you may not have any problem dating omnivores. If you're vegetarian strictly for health reasons, it may not bother you that your partner is eating meat. If you're vegetarian for moral reasons, however, you're going to have a hard time dating people who indulge in a practice that you find unethical.

It's no wonder that vegetarians often choose to only date other vegetarians. But that in itself brings its own set of drawbacks. For one thing, you're seriously limiting your dating pool. For another, what if you are dating a different kind of vegetarian than you are? To a vegan, even dating an ovo-lacto can cause problems.

If you do want to date other vegetarians, you'll have better luck if you live in a large metropolitan area. Many vegetarian societies have local groups that meet in larger towns and cities. Many of these groups have potluck get-togethers and outdoor events. There are also dating services just for vegetarians, as well as animal rights or animal welfare groups, and vegetarian cooking classes—all great places to meet vegetarian singles.

And don't rule out Internet dating. The number of people gravitating toward dating online grows all the time, and it's much more acceptable to meet potential mates this way than ever before. Sign up with a site that caters exclusively to vegetarian dating and, while you may not find as many members in the more all-inclusive services, you'll know from the start that you're meeting like-minded singles.

Vegetarianism at Work

If you've ever been on a weight-loss diet, you know what a royal pain co-workers can be. There's a strange sort of hive-mind mentality that happens in the workplace, where people simply can't accept that you don't want a piece of birthday cake or a piece of that giant submarine sandwich. Sometimes it's like being back in grade school—the peer pressure can be annoying, and it can sabotage your diet!

Vegetarians face a similar problem, especially if they're the only vegetarian eaters in their office. Sadly, it's human nature for people to feel threatened by any change in the status quo, and your becoming a vegetarian may cause people to become antagonistic, or to try and sway you to give up your commitment to a vegetarian lifestyle.

Even if you're polite and don't make a big deal out of your vegetarianism, it will most likely become an issue. "Come on ... just have one slice," they'll say when the pepperoni pizza is set out. "What are you now, some kind of hippy?" they'll ask. Usually they don't even know they're being rude and hostile; it will usually be presented in a joking manner. But it will be hard for you to stay cheerful if you find yourself continually under attack.

The best you can do is to smile, say, "No, thank you," in a calm voice, and change the subject. You may have to walk away if they don't drop the subject. But if the subject keeps coming up, perhaps you can use the situation to your advantage instead of becoming frustrated and angry. When they hit you with the usual jibes, come back with a clever response:

"I think tofu's disgusting."
"And eating a cow's liver isn't?"

"It's okay to eat animals, because humans are smarter."
"So does that mean it's okay to eat stupid people?"

"I'll bet one really great cheeseburger would change your mind."
"And I'll bet one trip to a slaughterhouse would change yours!"

"If you don't eat meat, why do you wear leather shoes?"
"Why? Are shoes made from meat?"

Besides the witty comebacks, when you begin to deal with someone who has the courage to ask a question like the last one, it's best to start with some common ground. For example, you may want to let them know that eating vegetarian saves quite a bit of water for the earth. Producing just a kilo of beef requires between thirteen thousand and hundred thousand liters of water, far more than you use for bathing in a single year. Given the current and expected water issues, it's not hard to see why this is such an issue. Eventually, fights over the rights to what little water is left on the planet are inevitable.

What's more, not only is nonvegetarianism a drain on water resources, but more than 50 percent of the world's forests have been cleared for cattle production alone. As a result, carbon dioxide plays into this equation as well. With rain forests being eliminated at record rates, carbon dioxide rates are out of control, and that's not only a real problem for people who live near the vanishing rain forests, but for all of us on a global level.

Keep in mind that the population of animals is exceedingly high already. There are seven billion people on the planet, but there are trillions of animals being raised to feed us. They are often forced to breed in a concurrent fashion (after they've given birth, they're inseminated again), and that only causes a more serious drain on the planet's resources as a whole. Each new birth, of course, means more food and water that's not being spent on the human population, and that leads to the world hunger problem that we see today. Because much of the grain resources are reserved for the richer nations, it never reaches the hungry mouths in third world countries.

Our own food choices determine the fate of people on a worldwide basis, and given that we're all interconnected, destruction in one nation ultimately means destruction in another. Once one given area goes down that we rely on for meat, agriculture, or something else, it's difficult, if not impossible, to replace it.

Because what we eat goes hand in hand with the overal health of the planet, going vegetarian or vegan for the sake of future generations as well as your health is really quite an important decision. Given that your choice can create either a positive or a negative effect for others, it's wise to consider all options. After all, just choosing to make others happy can make you happier in the long run.

In any case, starting with a common ground may help eliminate the useless debate that tends to occur in these situations. Showing a good sense of humor and ensuring that no one is antagonized or becomes defensive is the key. That applies to business functions like dinners with clients and conferences with catered lunches. If you're dining in a restaurant, all of the usual etiquette applies—eat what you can, or politely ask for something else. If you're stuck at a business function, however, and there's absolutely nothing to eat, share your vegetarianism with your boss or the person who plans your company's events. Once they start adding a vegetarian option to the fare at business meetings and other events, you'll find that you're not the only employee who enjoys that option; pretty soon you'll find that there's always something to eat at work.

CHAPTER 19

How to Create a Vegetarian Supportive Environment at Work and at Play

You now have a lot of valuable tools at your disposal—you know how to plan meals, you know what nutrients you need to keep your body healthy, and you know how to feed your vegetarian child. You even know how to answer questions from others and make sure you have plenty of healthful food to eat at home, at school, and at work.

Making your new lifestyle work at home and in the office requires a lot of flexibility, good humor, and planning. By this point though, you should feel up to the task. You've made excellent choices for your health and your future, and how you integrate them into the rest of your life will not only affect your relationships, but also how others view vegetarianism.

Nonvegetarians and Vegetarians—Managing a Mixed Marriage

All marriages are about compromise. You choose someone to spend the rest of your life with and, as time passes, you often find yourselves negotiating to find a middle ground that you can live with. One of you is messy, the other is neat. He loves reality television, she adores opera. One partner may be a social butterfly, but the other's happy to stay home every night with a good book. Married couples figure out how to adapt to such differences, and a vegetarian/nonvegetarian marriage has to negotiate many more obstacles than most.

It's understandable, when you're single and dating, to believe that the ideal partner will share all of your values. But that's unrealistic. No two individuals are exactly alike, and the day-to-day struggle of paying bills, doing laundry, getting to work, and raising children can sometimes make even the smallest difference seem enormous. As the popularity of vegetarianism increases, so do the number of mixed marriages between nonvegetarians and vegetarians. You and your spouse may agree on a lot of things, but still disagree on how to eat.

The key to making it work is acceptance of each other's choices. If you judge your spouse harshly for not joining you in your vegetarian journey, you may be turning them off entirely and closing the door to them making that step themselves in the future. No one likes to be told that they're going the wrong way, particularly if they're simply eating the same diet as most of the other people they see every day.

Try to keep in mind that your choice to become vegetarian was a personal one, and it has to be the same for them too. You can't control what your spouse eats, but you can control how you behave toward him or her.

Cherish the issues in your marriage that you agree on. There are probably far more of those than there are issues on which you don't see eye to eye.

Acknowledge that your spouse's diet isn't meant to hurt you. If your partner eats meat, it isn't a choice designed to make your life unhappy or more complicated. Try to respect his or her decision, whether it is based on ethical principles, on convenience, or on habit.

Try to get your partner to compromise on certain foods. See if you can get them to eat meat-free hot dogs, veggie burgers, and nondairy cheese at home.

Never attack your spouse's point of view, especially in public. Belittling your partner will only cause them to be resentful and more resistant to vegetarianism.

Try to find restaurants where you can eat together. Choose venues that offer both meat dishes and vegetarian options, so that you can enjoy a fine meal together.

Play an active role in shopping and preparing meals. Cook a variety of tasty, appealing meals so that your partner can see that the diet isn't boring. Buy a few cookbooks, and try new recipes to keep things interesting.

Be a positive role model. Allow your cheerful attitude and good health to serve as an example of how great vegetarianism can be.

Don't talk endlessly about your diet. If your partner is interested, the subject will come up naturally; don't lecture.

If you've agreed not to eat meat at home, accept that your spouse may eat meat sometimes when he or she is not with you. Again, you can't control what they eat, and nagging doesn't help.

Eating together is one of the greatest pleasures of any relationship. Negotiate a menu plan that's acceptable to both of you, and then enjoy your meals together!

Being Vegetarian at Work

If you work in a corporate environment, food is as much a part of your job as voicemail, computers, and fluorescent lighting. Lunch is where you network, make deals, and discuss contracts. Looking and acting professional in such situations is vital.

As a vegetarian, this can pose a unique challenge. If everyone around you is ordering steak or chicken Caesar salads and you're not eating much, it can call undue attention to your eating habits. Suddenly, no one's talking about the deal; they're talking about why you aren't eating your lunch!

More and more people are choosing vegetarian lifestyles, but that doesn't mean that being a vegetarian at work is easy. You've made a lifestyle choice dictated by your health and your ethics, but you have to walk the fine line of also fitting in with your colleagues. After all, if you're too independent a thinker, they might not believe that you're still a team player. When you're at work, you want the focus to be on your work, not on what you eat. The same grace, good humor, and tact that you use to deal with family and friends are even more important in the workplace.

Answering Questions and Looking Professional

Most of the time, nobody's going to care if you order a cheese omelet rather than ham and eggs. Sometimes, however, the comments made about what you ordered will be pointed, and they can even be just plain rude. If you've brought along a tempeh-and-pita sandwich and your colleague in the next cubicle tells you it looks disgusting, or if somebody at a power lunch says something insulting because you've ordered a hummus plate instead of a club sandwich, your best strategy is to simply act surprised that they care so much about what you eat. It deflects the obnoxious behavior and puts it in perspective. Why *do* they care so much about your food, anyway?

This is another situation in which you should be prepared to answer questions honestly but politely, while keeping your answers short. As we've mentioned already, you don't want the focus to be on your diet, nor do you want to come off as lecturing. At this point you should already know the answers to common questions, but let's review:

"So, what can you eat?" Tell them the truth, but downplay the tofu and tempeh. You can eat almost anything, after all, and if you tell them that, it'll put their minds at ease. "Most of the same things you eat—pizza, spaghetti, burritos—just without the meat," is always a good answer.

"Why did you become a vegetarian?" How you answer this depends on how well you know the person asking the question and how much personal detail you feel comfortable sharing with co-workers. Often, it's best to highlight the health benefits of vegetarianism. Sure, you could go into details about factory farming, the environment, and the ethics of eating sentient creatures, but most people will get your message more readily if you simply make it clear that you've found that eating a meatless diet is better for your health.

"Will it bother you if I eat meat?" Your co-workers will probably want to make sure you're comfortable, but often it's more about them—they want to know that they won't be judged if they continue to eat meat. The best way to get along with everyone is to respect their food choices and let them know that you aren't going to look down on them for eating meat. If you simply can't stand to be around people who are eating animal foods, find somewhere else to eat, but don't make a big deal out of it.

In every food-related situation that you find yourself in, you're an ambassador for vegetarianism. By maintaining the same calm, straightforward demeanor that you would in any professional situation, you'll go a long way toward educating people that there's nothing weird, boring, or threatening about the vegetarian lifestyle.

The Vegetarian Interview

When you are interviewing for a new position, you want to make the best impression possible. So what can you do when you are interviewing over lunch or dinner? What if you are invited out for a meal with your boss *and* prospective colleagues? Don't panic. You don't have to lie about being a vegetarian. There's nothing wrong about the way you choose to eat. So what if the rest of the party orders steak or hamburgers? They will admire your resolve for sticking to your vegetarian diet and not following the crowd. Just approach the situation in an honest, sincere, and genuine manner. Here are some tips:

Make a good first impression. Job interviews are all about first impressions. Let your future boss and/or colleagues focus on your strengths and assets in regard to work. If they ask you about your vegetarianism, answer their question and then shift the conversation back to the original position. You want the job to be the focus of the conversation, not the way you eat. That way, when they are assessing you at a later date, they will remember your abilities and confidence, and not the fact that you are a vegetarian.

Don't make it an issue. Being a vegetarian at work is a lot easier than people think. Don't make it into a problem. Let your prospective employer know that it's not an inconvenience and that you are willing to compromise in certain situations. For example, if the interview is taking place at a restaurant with limited vegetarian selections, don't complain. Simply do your best to find something to eat. Order soup and salad. Or, ask the waiter politely if a certain dish can be made according to your dietary needs. Handle the situation as professionally as possible. Your future boss will definitely take notice.

Make being a vegetarian into an asset. When you talk about being a vegetarian, highlight the reasons why you chose to change your diet. Talk about being healthier and more environmentally conscious, but not in a condescending way. Be confident and factual. Be open to answering any questions your boss or colleagues may have. Keep any personal views about nonvegetarians to yourself, however. You don't want to appear pompous and self-righteous. Don't get suckered into any political debates. Keep the conversation light and professional by adding in a bit of humor.

In the end, whether you get the job or not won't be determined by the food that you eat. If it is, then the job wasn't a right fit anyway. Would you really want to work for a company who hired you based on your eating habits? All you can do is put your best foot forward. If you get the job, you'll have to adjust to corporate meals and functions, and maintain the professional attitude you presented in the interview.

When Your Boss Foots the Bill

Part of corporate life is showing up for conferences, training sessions, and off-site meetings where food is ostensibly provided for you with a lot of thought. That thoughtfulness doesn't always extend to offering vegetarian options, however. Don't assume that vegetarian eaters will be catered to. If you know ahead of time that a corporate event is scheduled, by all means talk to your boss or to the employee in charge of planning the event and let them know you'd like a vegetarian meal. Usually, providing for vegetarians isn't a problem, but whoever's arranging for the food will need to know ahead of time how many vegetarian meals they would have to provide. If it's a big event, you're unlikely to be the only vegetarian!

If the planner is unfamiliar with vegetarian meals, offer some suggestions. Vegetable lasagna, spinach ravioli, Indian curries, eggplant Parmesan, vegetable burritos or hummus sandwiches are all dishes that can be made for a large number of people. If, for whatever reason, you're unable to get a vegetarian meal, as always, make do with what's on hand. Eat salad, bread, and side dishes. Even in the nicest restaurants or hotels, you can request a baked potato and a salad, and the kitchen will be happy to provide it for you.

Always remember that professional behavior is as important at the dining table as it is in the boardroom. If you throw a hissy fit about your lunch, you risk alienating your co-workers and looking bad in front of your superiors. No one wants to work with someone who's finicky, humorless, and inflexible, and that's precisely what your co-workers might think of you if you can't handle a single meal without throwing a tantrum.

Also keep in mind that while it may be perfectly acceptable to bring an alternate vegetarian dish to a friend's home when they throw a dinner party, bringing your own food to a corporate event is tacky. Even if there's nothing for you to eat except salad and bread sticks, put on a charming smile and eat what you can. Nobody said it would always be easy!

CHAPTER 20

Ethics, Beauty, and Health
Saving the Earth, One Veggie Burger at a Time

By now you've learned pretty much everything you need to know about becoming a vegetarian, from ethics to nutrition to meal planning. Just don't forget one of the biggest reasons that living a vegetarian lifestyle is a wonderful choice: what you eat affects the rest of the world.

Consider the effect of a nonvegetarian society on the planet:

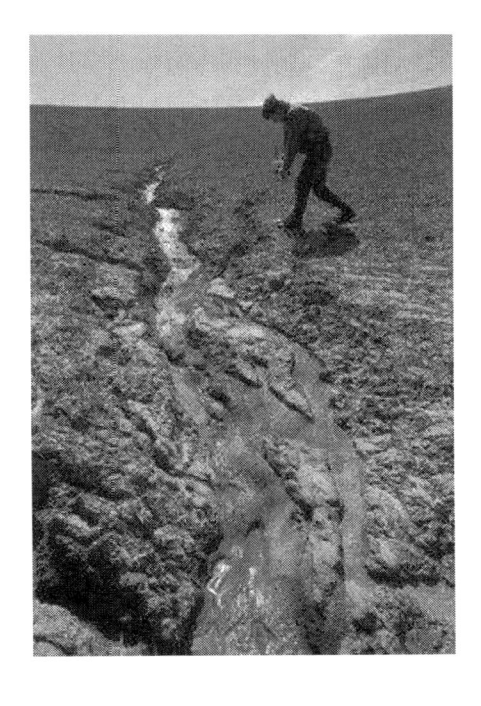

Water and soil damage. Two hundred and sixty million acres of U.S. forests have disappeared, to make room for cropland to farm meat. Producing one pound of beef requires at least 2,500 gallons of water. The manufacture of a single hamburger patty takes enough fossil fuel to drive a small car 25 miles. It takes less water to produce a year's worth of food for a vegetarian than to produce one month's food for a nonvegetarian. Factory farms damage the environment in addition to the horrors they commit on the animals that they raise and slaughter. They use large quantities of fossil fuels and fresh water, and pollute the earth in return.

In 2000, the World Commission on Water predicted that the increase in water use in the future due to rising population will "impose intolerable stresses on the environment, leading not only to a loss of biodiversity, but also to a vicious circle in which the stresses on the ecosystem will no longer provide the necessary services for plants and people." Ideas like that haven't disappeared nearly a decade later. By 2050, 59 percent of the world population will face some type of water shortage according to a 2009 study by the Stockholm Environment Institute.

Did you know that 85 percent American topsoil—over five billion tons—is lost annually due to the raising of livestock, and twenty-six billion tons of topsoil is lost annually on agricultural land worldwide? In the United States, one-third of the cropland has been permanently destroyed due to excessive soil erosion. By switching to a vegetarian diet, you alone spare an acre of trees every year.

Millions of acres of forests and wetlands have been leveled and drained to create pastures to feed the animals butchered for meat, destroying habitats for wildlife and disrupting the ecological balance. Irrigation of these pastures and croplands uses vast quantities of water, our most precious resource, and the water that runs off these lands takes with it irreplaceable topsoil, turning millions of acres of lush cropland into desert. Along with waste products from factory farming and slaughterhouses, runoff from agribusinesses contributes more pollution than all other human activities combined. The natural waste produced each year by the dairy cows in the 50-square-mile area of California's Chino Basin, for example, would make a pile with the dimension of a football field. When it rains heavily, dairy manure is washed straight down into the Santa Ana River and into the aquifer that supplies half of Orange County's drinking water.

A cultural shift toward vegetarianism would mean fewer animals in factory farms and feedlots, far less manure produced, and far cleaner water. It would also mean that our water would be healthier and far less likely to contain dangerous pathogens from animal waste. It would be a major step toward restoring the life-giving waters of our planet.

The choices we make directly affect our water supply, both on the earth and in our bodies. Every time you eat plant foods instead of meat, you are helping to reduce water pollution. Each of us is responsible for our own actions.

Depletion of rain forests. Between 1960 and 1985, nearly 40 percent of all Central American rain forests were destroyed to create pasture for beef cattle. That destruction, unfortunately, didn't end with the passing of the millennium. Experts now suggest the remaining rain forests will be eliminated over the course of the next forty years. As the primary source of oxygen for the entire planet, the survival of the rain forests is inextricably linked with the survival of mankind. The unique flora and fauna found in the rain forests provide ingredients for many medicines used to treat and cure human illnesses, and scientists are continuing to find new medicines as they discover new plants available only in these regions; yet approximately one thousand species go extinct every year due to destruction of tropical rain forests. By destroying the rain forests, we may be destroying the chance to cure AIDS, cancer, or influenza.

Poison in the atmosphere. The burning of fossil fuels creates two-thirds of carbon dioxide emissions worldwide, and two hundred gallons of fossil fuel are burned to produce the beef currently eaten by the average American family of four each year. Burning two hundred gallons of fossil fuel releases two tons of carbon dioxide into the atmosphere; by switching to a vegetarian diet, you're cutting back on the amount of pollution in the air. In 2001, the Intergovernmental Panel on Climate Change published a report that global warming was a much more serious issue than they had originally thought, five years previously. Newer reports indicate that the next century is likely to bring about a 2.7 to 11 degree change, causing massive alteration in weather patters and natural global disasters. Studies have shown that the year 2019 (which is right around the corner!) is the last turning point we can make to fight global warming. After that, the trend would be irreversible, which means complete disaster for mankind! The ice that is normally present in places like Greenland could melt completely. If Greenland ice does melt completely, it will increase sea level worldwide by at least seven meters, which would mean disaster to coastal cities like New York and Boston. The need for change in the way we eat and treat our planet has never been more urgent.

Poison in the workplace. The air inside factory farms contains a dangerous combination of ammonia, hydrogen sulfide, bacteria, and decomposing fecal matter. A joint study by the University of Iowa and the American Lung Association concluded that 70 percent of the workers in indoor facilities on factory pig farms experience symptoms of respiratory illness. Chronic bronchitis is suffered by over 50 percent of all swine confinement workers, which is three times that of farmers who work in outdoor facilities. The turnover rate of workers in these conditions is understandably very high, and in some cases, the owners of the factory farms have had to sell their businesses because they themselves were unable to work in their own farms.

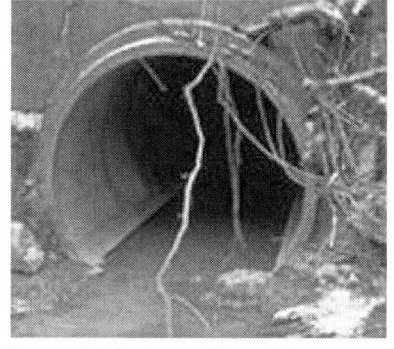

Consider this the next time you're complaining about your job: the decomposing waste from pigpens is collected in pits below, causing a build-up of hydrogen sulfide. According to the American Lung Association report, "Animals have died and workers have become seriously ill in confinement buildings. Several workers have died when entering a pit during or soon after the emptying process to repair pumping equipment. Persons attempting to rescue these workers have also died." The pigs living in these conditions breathe those toxic fumes every minute of their short lives. Animals living in these conditions regularly contract pneumonia and other respiratory illnesses—yet another reason why they're pumped full of antibiotics.

Economics. Raising animals for food is—to put it bluntly—a stupid way to feed a hungry world. Livestock in the United States consume enough grain and soybeans to feed more than five times the nation's population. One acre of pasture produces an average of 165 pounds of beef; the same acre could produce twenty thousand pounds of potatoes. If Americans reduced their consumption of meat by just 10 percent, it would save twelve million tons of grain annually. That much grain could feed sixty million people each year.

Eating Ethically

In reading this book, I hope that you've garnered some important ideas about why it makes good sense for your health and for the environment to live a vegetarian lifestyle. But there's another, very important reason: eating meat is, for lack of a better word, immoral.

All animals are living creatures with thoughts and emotions. They feel pain, just like you do. Vegans and vegetarians believe that animals are sensitive beings, not just things to be grown and slaughtered as we see fit. Vegans follow the strictest lifestyle in this regard and, even if you're not yet ready to take that path, it's worth considering the choices they make. Vegans don't eat anything from animal origin, including meat, eggs, dairy products, and honey. They don't wear leather or wool, and they don't use products made by companies that experiment on animals. They "walk the talk," as the saying goes, living by their principles and eschewing all products that involve the death and suffering of animals.

Every year, billions of animals—sensitive, sentient beings that feel intense pain and suffering — are transformed into food products in a world where we can very easily get all the nutrition we need from plant foods. Their misery is completely unnecessary. We do not need to kill animals to live, we kill animals simply because we believe we have the right to do so. Vegans and vegetarians can't stop these atrocities from happening, but they can refuse to participate in the process.

It's no coincidence that many of the world's great religions have espoused vegetarianism as part of the journey to enlightenment. There are stories of great spiritual leaders who had the road in front of them gently swept as they walked so that they wouldn't accidentally step on an insect on the road. Some spiritually advanced Yogis have evolved their morals to the point where they can't bear to swat a mosquito. The progress of moral values is a long evolution, begun when a small minority of people adopted values which would eventually be adopted by the rest of society. If you have natural empathy for animals and if you can't bear to eat their flesh, then live by the courage of your convictions; display your feelings and empathy for animals by refusing to contribute to their suffering.

Beautiful Inside and Outside

Eating a vegetarian diet will help you live longer, as you're avoiding foods that create free radicals in your system which hasten the aging process. You'll look younger longer because of this, and your skin and hair will glow with good health. But the biggest beauty benefit is the one that comes from within—the radiance that comes from living an ethical, more spiritual life.

You don't have to be religious to be spiritual. You don't even have to believe in any sort of divine power. But take a moment to think about the connection between the great religions and respect for animals.

There's a reason that so many people who are concerned about man's warring nature are also vegetarians. When you are conscious that animals have souls—that they're alive, and conscious, and feel pain—how can you kill them unnecessarily? If you believe that animals think and feel and suffer, then you believe in the soul and, therefore, that all living things are spiritual in essence.

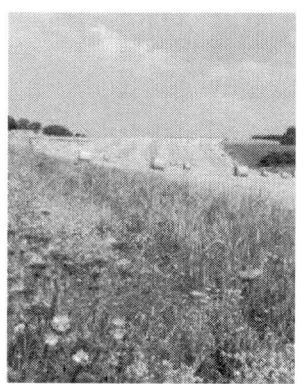

On a more pragmatic note, animals are tortured in terrible ways in slaughterhouses. Pigs scream in fear, often dropping dead due to heart attack because of the terror they experience on the killing floor. The adrenalin produced in these animals' bodies when they're under such intense stress permeates every part of them, producing toxins that are passed on into the animal products that nonvegetarians consume. People who eat meat produced under such conditions can't help but be affected by them—and they, in turn, interact with the people around them while these substances are in their own bodies.

The Karma Connection

Some Buddhists, who believe in the concept of karma, are not vegetarians. It's certainly recommended for them to avoid eating meat, but not required. Many Buddhists around the world choose a vegetarian lifestyle, though, because they feel strongly that it connects to the laws of karma.

In a nutshell, karma is the concept that what goes around comes around. If, as individuals, we want to bring peace, harmony, and unity to the world, it simply doesn't make sense to contribute to the world's violence by killing animals. Violence breeds violence, whether it's the killing of animals, muggings in the street, murders, or wars between nations. The Nobel Prize winner Isaac Bashevis Singer once asked, "How can we pray to God for mercy if we ourselves have no mercy? How can we speak of rights and justice if we take an innocent creature and shed its blood? I personally believe that as long as human beings will go on shedding the blood of animals, there will never be any peace."

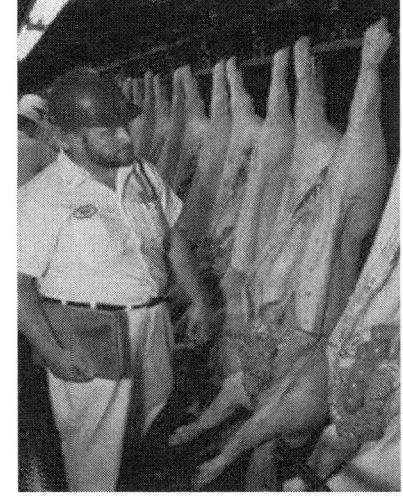

Buddhists believe that we affect and are affected by a collective karma. Karma works like a spiritual bank account—if you've caused bad karma, you'll be reborn as a lesser being, like an animal or a demon. If you live a moral life, however, and spread good karma during your time on earth, you'll be reborn as a human—or even, should you attain enlightenment, a Buddha. The Buddha once said, "... if in the process of repayment, the lives of other beings were taken or their flesh eaten, then it will start a cycle of mutual devouring and slaughtering that will send the debtors and creditors up and down endlessly."

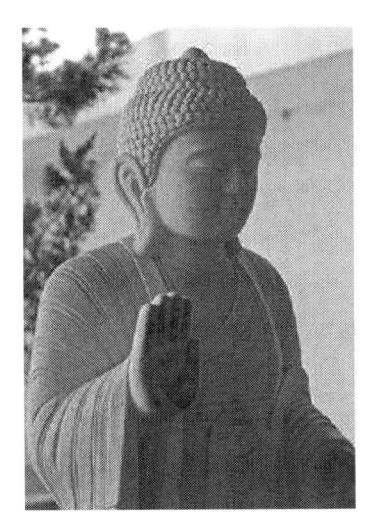

As one story goes, a disciple of the Buddha asked a man why he kept buying meat from the butcher. The man replied that he bought meat because the butcher kept selling meat. So the disciple then asked the butcher why he sold meat, and the butcher answered that he did so because the man kept buying it. The Buddha said that both men were lacking in compassion and wisdom.

Supply and demand is the foundation of economy. The cycle of meat consumption and animal slaughtering is a complex network of interdependence. By becoming a vegetarian, you're doing your part to stop the violence.

Making Healthy Food Choices for the Planet

Everything—every animal, plant, and person—is interconnected. What you choose to eat not only affects your body, it affects the planet and every living thing on it as well. We may believe that it is the economy that provides us with food, air, water, and energy. The truth is that it's the earth that provides us with all of these things. And if we continue to abuse the earth in such a way, those things that we have taken for granted will eventually cease to exist. We will undermine our own survival if we continue to pollute the air and water, destroy natural rain forests, and produce destructive greenhouses gasses. Thankfully, an environmental awareness movement is taking place. People are more aware of how they treat the planet, and this includes what they choose to eat.

Consider this: is a quarter pound of hamburger worth a half ton of Brazil's rain forest? Or perhaps 67 square feet of rain forest is a little too much to pay for one hamburger. Put in that context, that one hamburger pales in comparison. We need the earth's forests more than we need a hamburger fix. They are the source of oxygen for every life on the planet. They regulate our climates, prevent floods, and check soil erosion. They recycle and purify our water. They provide wood for paper and buildings and fires. We need our forests to survive. Recycling is only half of the battle. Cutting down meat consumption from cattle farms and the like, is the other half.

If we eat less meat, the majority of land out west in the United States could be used as a sustainable, environmentally friendly resource, rather than for cattle farming. Large solar energy and wind-power facilities could be built instead, generating enormous amounts of energy without the side effect of pollution. Land that isn't used could serve as a natural wildlife refuge and habitat. Any shift toward a vegetarian lifestyle would have an immense positive impact, not only on the country but also on the world. Life would continue for many species on the cusp of extinction.

The Future for Food, People, and Earth

There is far more at stake here than some people care to realize. Becoming a vegetarian is only a key element to the overall picture. Whether we embrace what is occurring or not, the choices we make (as individuals and as a whole) will have a profound effect on the future of our species and on earth. When you make the choice to respect the food on our planet, you are choosing to help uphold the spirit, natural beauty, and interconnectedness of the earth. You become an integral part in the preservation of all life forms and will help to build a healthier and more sustainable future for generations to come.

Unfortunately, we do not have the luxury of time to turn things around for our planet and our human race. According to many scientific research studies, and a documentary called *Home*, we have only until 2019 before we pass the point of no return. This means that we have to act now. Every time you choose to eat plant-based foods instead of meat, you are making a conscious choice to help the environment. It is as if you are taking the time to plant trees every day of your life in order to create a greener and a much healthier future for life everywhere. Choosing to eat consciously now will allow the children of the future to learn to live harmoniously with the natural ecosystems of the world. We can save the world, one vegetarian at a time.

CHAPTER 21

The Path Ahead
Enjoying Your Vegetarian Lifestyle for the Rest of Your Life

Congratulations! If you've followed all the steps and taken the advice presented to you in this book, you're a vegetarian! Now you have one more decision to make: whether or not you want to use your knowledge to reach out to other vegetarians and educate nonvegetarians about the vegetarian lifestyle. You don't have to do this, of course. You can live your vegetarian life quietly and on your own, and there's nothing wrong with that. But now that you know what you do about vegetarianism's value to individuals and the world, you may find you want to become a bit more active.

You don't have to do it right this minute, of course. But many, many vegetarians find that it's easier to maintain their lifestyle if they have the support of others who share the same values. As you now know, there are many reasons for becoming vegetarian, and people have all sorts of different reasons for making the switch; and you may find that there's a lot to learn by discovering the viewpoint of other vegetarians.

Even if you choose to travel this path alone, you're an ambassador for vegetarianism. Your family, friends, co-workers, and even strangers will see you as an example of meatless living, and as you meet more people and have more unique experiences of your own, your outlook, appearance, and behavior will—for better or worse—be seen as that of a vegetarian person. So, why not become the best vegetarian that you can be?

First Impressions

Whether we like it or not, our appearance and actions are judged by others. If you're telling a co-worker about the barbaric treatment of cows in factory farms while eating a cheese sandwich or discussing karma and you're wearing leather shoes, your audience may see you as a hypocrite. That's not to say that you can't be a good vegetarian and eat cheese or wear leather, but that you need to be aware of when your actions and your words aren't in alignment.

Always practice good hygiene and dress neatly. Don't play into society's prejudices by exemplifying the stereotype of the dirty hippy. If you're clean, neat, and appropriately dressed, the people that you deal with will think, "Hey, you're just like me!" They'll hear your message because they relate to you, rather than being turned off due to their own preconceptions.

Making the Connection

If you live in a small town, it may be difficult for you to find other vegetarians to talk to about the lifestyle. But don't give up! If you have a college or university in your town, there's probably a vegetarian group on campus—higher education and vegetarianism often go hand-in-hand. Watch for notices of vegetarian group meetings posted on bulletin boards at colleges, schools, and community centers, as well as libraries, supermarkets, and other public places. Check out the ads in your local newspaper and look for natural food stores, bookstores, or other shops that support alternative lifestyles. Visit them, and ask questions; in a small town, word of mouth is invaluable.

The Internet is also a great resource for vegetarians. There are hundreds of online groups, including message boards and recipe-swap sites, geared toward vegetarians. Not only are they a good source of discussion and community, they may be able to connect you with vegetarians in your own area. If you aren't aware of it, Seventh-Day Adventists are vegetarian, so if there's a vegetarian group in your area, the church probably knows about it.

If you still find yourself coming up short, take the initiative and start your own group! It's highly unlikely that you're the only vegetarian where you live, even in a rural area or a very small town. Take out a newspaper ad and throw a potluck at your home or local community center. You may be pleasantly surprised by how many people show up! Once you've got a group together, start a regular event where you all eat out at local restaurants. You'll not only help your community by supporting restaurants that cater to vegetarian diners, you may also encourage other local businesses to take vegetarians into consideration when planning their menus.

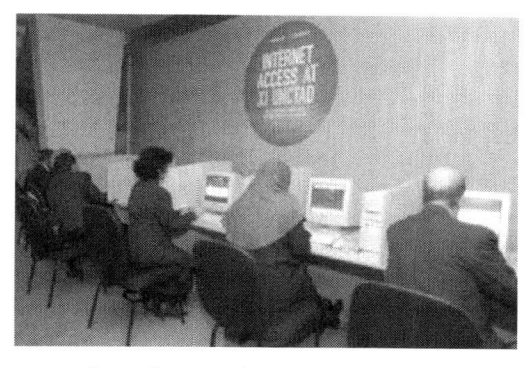

As a newcomer to vegetarianism, you'll probably find it helpful to socialize with others who share your point of view. Even the most well-meaning friends can be less than supportive of a lifestyle change, because they think they already know who you are and what you like. But by making connections with others who feel the same way, you'll not only broaden your own social network, you'll have a valuable resource for asking questions, sharing ideas, and learning about other approaches to vegetarian eating.

Getting Active

As you've learned more about the ethical reasons for becoming a vegetarian, you may find yourself wanting to do something a bit more proactive—like joining an animal rights organization or working to promote meat-free eating in your community. The fist step is to assess how you'll fit this into your already busy life. If you have a full-time job and a family, you're already struggling to make time for your partner, your friends, your work, and your leisure activities. Do you have time to devote to activism? Take a hard look at all the responsibilities you juggle, and figure out how much of your day-to-day chores you can shift to your spouse, co-workers, and others to allow you time for activism.

One way to manage this is to try and incorporate activist activities into the existing areas of your life. You can share a video on factory farming practices with your church group, for example, or ask your employer if they would consider supporting an animal rights organization at a local event.

Always pick your battles carefully. There are a lot of terrible things going on in the world, and you're just one person. It's better to make a real difference on one issue than to spread yourself so thin that you're ineffective at all of them. Your activism could be as simple as starting a vegetarian support group or helping out at an animals rescue group, or as intensive as becoming a full-time PETA volunteer. But choose your fight, and devote yourself fully to it.

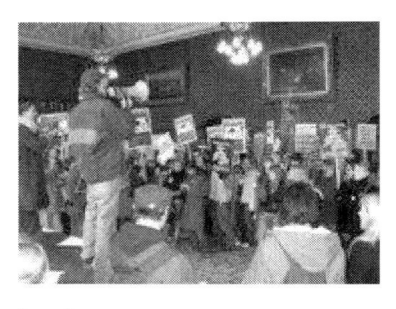

The important thing is to think carefully about how you can realistically work activism into your life. You're going to be a vegetarian for years, and excited as you may be right now to jump into serious activism, if you burn yourself out by adding even more activities to a busy life, you'll be shortchanging yourself and everyone else. You have a lot of time; do what you can, when you can, and you're still doing a lot more to help the world than most people!

Consider Other Ways You Can Go Green Once

Once you start eating ethically, it's a short hop to thinking about your other habits that harm the earth. You may not want to adopt a 100 percent sustainable lifestyle—and, frankly, in today's world, it's almost impossible to do so—but there are a number of ways that you can lessen your impact on the environment in addition to your vegetarian lifestyle:

Reduce, reuse, recycle. When you buy new products, ask yourself: Do I really need this? Is there another product which would do the same thing but with less impact on the environment? Will this last a long time? Are the materials used to make this renewable? Buy items that are durable, maintain them, and have them repaired if possible. If you don't need something that's taking up space in your home, give it to someone who does! And recycle whenever possible to cut down on matter going to landfills.

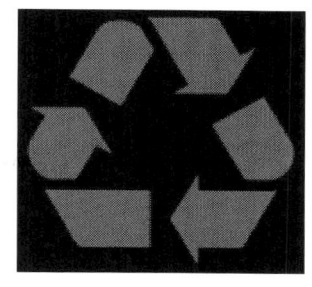

Treasure your resources, and cut back on waste. Fix your leaky faucets, toilets, or water pipes, and install water-saving faucets. Conserve fuel by turning down the heat at night and when you're away from your home, or install a programmable thermostat. Insulate your home against heat loss, and periodically check insulation. Avoid driving; walk, cycle, or use public transportation whenever possible. Use recycled batteries for appliances that require them. Buy locally; it's good for the local economy, and it saves energy because it hasn't traveled far to get to you.

Use less toxic substances in your home. Use nontoxic cleaning alternatives in your home. Buy furniture made from natural fibers, wood, metal, and glass. Avoid the use of polyvinyl chloride (PVC) in your home, including shower curtains, flooring, and children's toys. Avoid the use of aerosol sprays.

Be responsible with your waste. Don't put toxic household wastes such as paint, paint thinner, and antifreeze in the garbage or down the drain. Check with your local waste facility for proper disposal. Take your own bags to the grocery store, and use plastic bags until they're completely worn out. Avoid excess packaging, and always use reusable products rather than disposable ones—plates, napkins, mugs, lunch containers, batteries, pens, and razors.

Go green at work. Print on both sides of the paper you use, and reduce the number of copies you print. Buy recycled, chlorine-free paper, and have a recycling box under your desk for used paper goods. Buy a permanent mesh coffee filter instead of buying disposable paper filters. Encourage your workplace to use alternative cleaning materials. Use refillable pens and pencils rather than disposable ones. Walk, ride a bike, use public transit, or carpool to work.

Conserve in the kitchen. Your refrigerator uses more energy than any other appliance in your home, so try to keep energy use to a minimum. Keep the temperature of the main body between 38–42°F and that of the freezer at 0–5°F. Open the refrigerator door less frequently, and clean the condenser coils at least once a year. Use electric kettles to boil water—they use half the energy as boiling water on the stove. Avoid storing food in plastic; use reusable glass containers for storing food in the refrigerator. Never microwave food in a plastic container; even microwavable plastics can leech chemicals into your food when heated. Buy food in bulk whenever possible, as it's cheaper and uses less packaging. Look for products made from recycled materials, and use cloth instead of paper napkins and towels.

You're On Your Way!

Thomas Edison once said, "Nonviolence leads to the highest ethics, which is the goal of all evolution. Until we stop harming all other living beings, we are still savages."

You've made a wise decision by choosing a vegetarian lifestyle. Enjoy the new world of interesting foods that you'll discover, and be proud of yourself for taking an ethical, responsible path through life's great journey. It will be a fulfilling and healthful adventure that you'll enjoy for years to come. You will look back at this decision and be glad that you made it!

You realize that instead of spending your money on hospital bills, you can enjoy your golden years with your loved ones with great vitality! Not so many people are this fortunate!

You realize that the planet is in better shape because of your decision. You can look at younger generations in the eyes, without saying, "I'm sorry I made this mess."

You realize that more food and water is available for humans because of your decision. And they're grateful for it. So are the animals!

You just know that you made a really good decision. And you can't hold your smiles every time this comes to your mind. It's a victory for you, your loved ones, the planet, and the animals. And I want to congratulate you for that.

Congratulations, my friend!

Sincerely,

Rudy Hadisentosa

CHAPTER 22

FAQ

Finding the Answers to the Most Commonly Asked Questions about Vegetarianism

Many people have e-mailed me with questions ranging from general to specific. Below, I've included some of those questions. Each question contains a brief answer as well as an indication as to which chapter in the book you can go to in order to find more detailed information. My goal in writing this book was to offer you a genuine and feasible reason to switch to vegetarianism and give you the keys on how to make the transition as easy as possible. I hope you have enjoyed this book as much as I enjoyed writing it. But more importantly, I hope I have given you many reasons to become a vegetarian.

Q. *My child is fourteen years old and recently decided to become a vegetarian. How can I be sure that they will grow up healthy and strong?*

A. Getting all the vitamins, nutrients, and protein your body requires as a vegetarian adolescent is a lot easier than people think. Read chapter 17 for more information on raising healthy vegetarians.

Q. *How do you know if food contains dairy or meat?*

A. It's not always easy to know whether the food you are eating contains dairy or meat products, especially if you don't cook the meal yourself. Browse chapter 8 for more information on identifying hidden animal products.

Q. *What do I buy at the grocery store besides salad for vegetarian meals?*

A. There are far more food options for vegetarians than people think. Browse chapter 12 for more information on stocking your meatless kitchen with healthy, tasty, and nutritional vegetarian items.

Q. *How can I be sure that my body is getting everything it needs on a vegetarian diet?*

A. This is probably one of the biggest concerns for people who convert to vegetarianism. You can easily get everything your body needs (even protein!) on a vegetarian diet. Just take a glance at chapter 5, and brush up on vegetarian nutrition.

Q. *Can I lose weight on a vegetarian diet?*

A. There are many different reasons why people choose to become vegetarians. One of those reasons is to live a healthier lifestyle and lose weight. Browse chapter 10 for key tips on how to lose weight and balance your eating habits on a vegetarian diet. You can also take a look at chapter 11 to read up on the importance of exercise.

Q. *What do I do if I crave meat?*

A. Sticking to a vegetarian diet can be hard for those individuals who are just starting out on their vegetarian lifestyle. For tips and advice on how to stay on track, take a look at chapter 4 on how to get started on your journey and at chapter 8 on how to avoid setbacks, find support, and resist cravings.

Q. *I'm a high school student and a vegetarian. What can I do about eating lunch in the cafeteria?*

A. Maintaining your vegetarian lifestyle at school and/or at work can be somewhat of a challenge, especially if your food options are limited. Browse chapter 9, and you'll find ways to enjoy vegetarian options at restaurants, on the road, at work, *and* in the school cafeteria!

Q. *How can I make vegetarian meals that taste good?*

A. There is a common misconception that all vegetarian meals are tasteless. This couldn't be further from the truth. Browse chapter 13 for some great (and delicious!) vegetarian recipes to get you started!

Q. *How can I stay an active and competitive athlete on a vegetarian diet?*

A. Athletic vegetarians are often concerned about not being able to perform at a high level without the added protein from meat and eggs. Take a look at chapter 16 on how to eat well and be active at the same time. There are vegetarian athletes all over the world!

Q. *How can I get my whole family involved?*

A. Involving your entire family can be a bit of a challenge. When it's just you, sticking to a vegetarian lifestyle is much easier. But when you have a spouse and/or kids to think about, you have to be able to compromise. Browse chapters 8 and 17 for tips about coping in a meat-eating family and raising a family on a vegetarian diet.

Q. *Is drinking milk against vegetarian principles, and are dairy products good or bad?*

A. No, there are vegetarians who still eat dairy products. For more information about the pros and cons of dairy, take a look at chapter 15. I would advise you to stay away from dairy products whenever possible. If you're just starting out, it's okay to consume it sometimes, but later your body will learn to reject dairy because it's just not for human consumption! That's the reason why vegans don't consume dairy products either.

Q. *How do you make your co-workers accept your vegetarianism?*

A. Managing your vegetarianism at work can be tricky. Read up on this and other social/work situations in chapter 19. You can learn how to create a support environment both at home and at the office.

Q. *What does it really mean to be a vegetarian, and how will it benefit my overall health?*

A. Being a vegetarian will not only be healthy for you physically, it will also be healthy for you on a mental, spiritual, and emotional level. Read chapter 2 to gain a better understanding about the history of vegetarianism. Then, read chapter 3 to learn how being a vegetarian is not only beneficial to you but also to our planet. Chapter 7 will also give you a better understanding on how you will be a healthier and happier individual by becoming a vegetarian.

Q. *What if I want to have my family and friends over for a holiday meal? As a vegetarian, how can I cook something that we all can enjoy?*

A. Holiday meals present a great opportunity to experiment with different vegetarian recipes. Read chapter 18 to learn more about planning dinner parties with friends or cooking a holiday meal that the whole family is sure to enjoy. You'll quickly see that it's not as difficult as you may think!

Q. *Are soy products bad for you?*

A. Soy products have been the subject of many scientific studies lately, and the results are not good. While tempeh is fine to eat in moderation, other soy products (like soy milk) should not be consumed on a regular basis. Read chapter 14 to learn more about soy products and why you should avoid them and choose other meat alternatives instead.

Q. *How do I deal with this argument from a friend: If we don't kill the animals, there would be too many of them, and they will roam the world!*

A. The reason why there are now trillions of animals in our planet is because we made them. The cows are inseminated again right after they have done giving birth; if humans are treated this way, each family would have probably twenty to thirty children. No wonder there are so many animals on this planet. The same applies to chicken, fishes, ducks, pigs, and all meat-factory animals.

Remember, our resources are being used on them, instead of on humans. The more animals there are, the less we can use our resources to solve our planet's problems.

Q. *Whatever the question is ...*

A. Always answer the question with a common ground, using examples such as the water problem that we are currently facing in this world and the changing climate that comes down hard on food production and adversely affects our future. Explain that meat industry is one of the most destructive industries on the planet because it clears more than 50 percent forests around the world. A major portion of the world's crops are being fed to animals instead of humans.

You can also explain how going vegetarian could save people's lives and help them avoid huge hospital bills. Looking at the statistics, it is clear that if we do what others do, we will end up like them. Only by changing our diet is it possible to avoid becoming one of the statistics.

If you explain it like this, the listener would have to agree with you because there's nothing that they can debate on. Never start with the issue of killing or not killing animals because if you do so, people can get aggressive.

Actually, even as vegans, we kill animals all the time. There are thousands of insects and other small animals that get killed in the process by which we get our fruits, vegetables, and other natural foods. The most we can do is just minimize the killings, but not stop it altogether. It's impossible to live without somehow killing small living beings. Therefore, don't use the above argument.

Answer in a way that creates mutual understanding between you and your listener. By explaining the health benefits they would get by eating more fruits and vegetables, you are helping them to live healthier and be less vulnerable to chronic diseases. They'll be thankful to you as long as you answer any questions they have in a nonjudgmental way. Nobody likes to be judged! Nor should we presume to do so!

Remember that every time you answer questions about being a vegetarian, you are actually making others' lives much better, for many people don't know that what they consider their "normal" diet is actually harming them!

So be happy about it!

You're making a difference in almost every new person you meet. What a *huge* blessing it is when you think about it!

So smile—because you deserve it.

Enjoy!

Rudy Hadisentosa

About the Author

Hello there

I am Rudy Hadisentosa, and I want to thank you for taking the time to read my book. It is a great pleasure for me to see you decide to become a vegetarian. It is a decision that you'll never regret in your whole life!

So congratulations!

A little about me:

I grew up in a small town called Bandarlampung, in Indonesia. I spent eighteen years there before I went to the United States for college. I joined the Ohio State University and graduated in 2004. After graduation, I went back to Indonesia and am now currently living in Jakarta.

With time, I realized that, just like me, a lot of people have a really tough time in becoming vegetarian. In 2006, I decided to launch a nonprofit Web site, www.veggie123.com, and offer my e-book free on it to help them make the changeover. You can also get some further health tips on the site by subscribing to the newsletter. The Web site is newly designed, and I'm starting a blog too. Please subscribe to my RSS.

I hope to be able to spread vegetarianism as much as possible because the world really needs it, and I think you do too. We all are in this together. We only have one planet to live in, don't we? So let's work hard to make a better future for younger generations. If we all work together, surely we can make a difference.

Though the vegetarian trend is gaining momentum, we need to spread it faster, or else this planet will be uninhabitable someday.

Let's all work together.

Rudy

Printed in Poland
by Amazon Fulfillment
Poland Sp. z o.o., Wrocław